D1333740

Diet, De-Stress, Detox

The Formula For Reclaiming Your Health & Vitality

By Kevin W. Reese

Library of Congress Control Number: 2014912273

Seven Thirty Enterprises LLC

PO Box 380261

East Hartford, CT 06138

ISBN: 0692240594

ISBN-13: 978-0692240595

Disclaimer

Nothing written in this book should be viewed as a substitute for competent medical care. This book, with the opinions, suggestions, and references made within it, is based on the author's personal experience and is for personal study and research purposes only. This program is about health and vitality, not disease. If you choose to use the material in this book on yourself, the author and publisher take no responsibility for your action and decision or the consequences thereof. It is encouraged that you take responsibility for yourself and search for your own truth in your wellness journey.

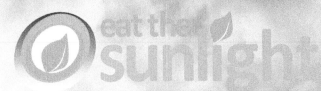

eat the sunlight

THIS BOOK WAS CREATED FROM EXPERIENCE

KEVIN W. REESE

Was Sick of Visiting His MD,
So He Took Control Back!

- ✓ Quit Smoking
- ✓ Overcame Anxiety
- ✓ Beat Insomnia

- ✓ Reversed Acid Reflux
- ✓ Learned How To De-Stress
- ✓ Lost Nearly 80 Pounds

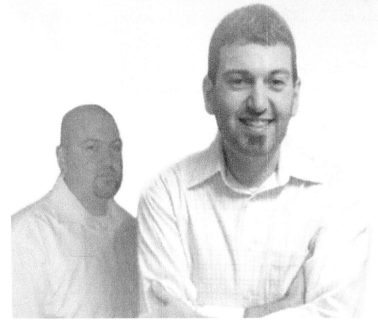

What's Free on
www.EATTHESUNLIGHT.com

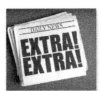

DAILY BLOG
Log on daily and stay up to date with the worlds Holistic Health News. Also receive the TOP 5 STORIES AND TIPS every Monday by signing up for our Newsletter.

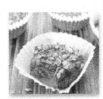

RECIPES
Everyone can add Sunlight! With a massive selection of both RAW and COOKED dishes, every recipe is Meat, Dairy, Egg, Gluten, and Soy FREE.

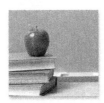

EDUCATIONAL LIBRARY
We did the research for you! We grouped together eye-opening videos and articles on such topics as GMO's, Vaccinations, Cancer, Juicing, and more.

SUNLIGHT RAPS
Founder, Kevin W. Reese merges Health & Hip-Hop as he performs Rap verses on Apples, Celery, Cucumbers and more. These videos are entertaining & educational for you or the kids!

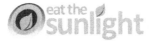

PUBLISHED WORKS

By Kevin W. Reese

Diet, De-Stress, Detox:

The Formula For Reclaiming Your Health & Vitality

Root Cause:

The Liberating Truth Behind Chronic Illness

Protein Kills:

Seven Reasons Why a High-Protein Diet Can Be Deadly

KevinWReese.com

Dedication

This book is dedicated to the clients who took a chance on me early in my health career. If it wasn't for the belief you had in me, this book would not be possible. I can't imagine it was easy to take a "shock jock" radio host seriously, but you did. Because of that, I had the opportunity for my theories and methods to be put to use which created the foundation to this book. I am grateful to have worked with you.

HASHTAGS

With social media and hash tags a worldwide standard these days, I wanted to design a way where we can all inspire and support each other interactively. I did this by placing "social media assignments" throughout the book. Now, all we have to do is look up the hash tags and find others taking the same journey. I hope you will participate.

#ThreeDLife

#EatTheSunlight

CONTENTS

ACKNOWLEDGMENTS

I want to acknowledge the natural health practitioners, researchers, experimenters, teachers, coaches, and healers that came before me. Very brave people like Ehret, Shelton, Tildon, Gandhi, Just, Hotema, Bragg, Walker, Brandt, Burroughs, Christopher, Lalanne, Graham, Cousins, Siegel, Gerson, Campbell, Rosenthal, Wolfe, McDonald, Meyerowitz, Sebi, Jensen, and Morse. Each of their work has contributed to what true health and vitality is.

CHAPTER 1
THE PROBLEM AND THE SOLUTION

SICK SOCIETY

As a Chronic Illness Specialist and Health Coach, I speak to many people who are suffering. They're in pain, they're unhappy, and they're confused. They don't understand why their medical doctor (MD) has no solution for them. They're sick of taking pills, they're sick of no answers, and they're sick of not knowing what to do.

I recently spoke to a woman in her early 40's whose IBS (Irritable Bowel Syndrome) is so bad she's bedridden. Her life is completely upside down as she can only leave the house in between frequent flare-ups. These flare-ups are so frequent and painful that she now has high anxiety due to the thought of a flare-up happening in public. Her MDs have no clue what to do. They have informed her that her suffering is permanent, and all she can do is relieve the pain with medication. But here is the catch: No meds have worked yet! So, for the last year, her MDs have been testing medicines on her to find one that relieves the pain. So essentially, she's a guinea pig.

I spoke to another young lady a few weeks ago, who has had Lupus since she was sixteen! (She is now thirty-two.) And get this: She now has tumors in her brain. Her MDs performed brain surgery. Almost a year later, they had to do another surgery. She had to train her young seven-year-old to call 911 just in case "mommy gets sick." So with a young child at home, and living far away from her immediate family, she told me she refuses to go through a third surgery.

Another woman I recently spoke to had a cyst on her pancreas. I advised her to do my program so we could reverse the cause, but the medical establishment had her so scared, she opted to go their route. So a few weeks later, they rushed her into surgery, removed her spleen, and a chunk of the pancreas to avoid "cancer." I followed up with her after the surgery to see how she was doing, and she said it was the worst experience of her life.

All three examples I gave are just the tip of the iceberg of what I hear from people on a weekly basis. People are suffering now more than ever, and it's happening to folks under the age of forty at a rapid rate. Cancer has tripled since 1980, two-thirds of Americans are overweight, and half are taking prescription pills for chronic issues. Yet, we have the technology to stream live videos from our Smartphones and send men to outer space.

These chronic illnesses (CIs) don't fall from the sky. You don't catch arthritis, type 2 diabetes, or lupus by drinking out of a public water fountain. It's not malaria. It's not the bubonic plague. It's simply malfunctions of the body that have manifested over time.

IS HELP POSSIBLE?

Chronic Illnesses are caused by poor lifestyle choices. This is why your MD can't do anything for you. He or she is not trained to reverse the root cause—they're trained to treat symptoms with medicine. This is why they are called "medical" doctors. The root meaning of medical is medicine. They are medics, and medics treat symptoms. And in treating you, they make a lot of money off of prescribing you pills. Yes, your MD makes money off that. In fact, some get bonuses, vacations, concert tickets, and more. They have invested interest.

I respect the talent of medics and nurses, especially in the case of an emergency. They have to work under stressful situations, and we should salute them. But I think we should be honest with ourselves and start seeing medics for what their specialty is. They're trained to handle acute and immediate cases. In other words, if you're having an asthma attack, a stroke, or you need your appendix taken out, I can't do anything for you, but a medic or nurse can! But if you have fibromyalgia, lupus, or migraine headaches, a CI Specialist can reverse your situation, while the medic or nurse can only ease your pain with medicine. Make sense? There's a difference between acute and chronic. And certainly, there are differences between a medical doctor and a CI Specialist.

A CI Specialist, such as myself, is a holistic health coach with expertise in the physiological mechanisms behind chronic conditions of the human body, and practical training in how natural foods and stress management techniques target and eliminate the root cause of these conditions. We assess your unique situation and create a customized protocol that harnesses the power of natural foods and detoxification to clean and strengthen your body and inspire the restoration of your glands, organs, and cells.

CI Specialists are experienced with the following issues:

-Arthritis   -Fibromyalgia

-Lupus   -Eczema

-High Blood Pressure   -Migraines

-Crohn's   -IBS

-Diverticulitis   -Endometriosis

-Fibroids   -Type 2 Diabetes

-Colitis   -COPD

As you read this, you may not have a chronic illness. But, if you're eating poorly, stressed to the core, and do not clean your insides…you will! Maybe even two. How can I be so sure? Well, forget my training or experience—it's just flat out common sense. If you go 100 mph on the highway everyday while checking your text messages, eventually you're going to have an accident. You may not feel it at fifteen, you may not even feel it at twenty-five, but watch what happens at or before forty! And fifty? Your MD will put you on pills, and you will live an artificial life, which will get worse with time. Eventually it manifests into cancer in your sixties, seventies, or eighties.

Cancer is what usually happens after the chronic phase. Chronic turns to degenerative because your acids and wastes are pressing up against the cells for a long period of time. One must understand, the same things that cause a CI caused the cancer. Like a CI, you can't "catch" cancer from touching a railing after someone sneezed on it. It's not a virus. It's another malfunction of the body manifested over time. The medical establishment will scare you into getting expensive treatment, but that treatment will NOT reverse the cause! This is why most people who get treatment and "beat" the "disease" get cancer again five to ten years later in another area of the body. Of course the medical establishment refers to this as "spreading." I assure you, nothing spread! They just never fixed the problem; they only treated the symptom. A "cancerous" tumor is only a symptom of a root cause, just as a fever is only a symptom of a root cause.

We must wake up and start focusing on the cause. For every cause, there is an effect. We often gather together and do "walks for the cure" type events, when we should be marching for the cause. Humans know how to unite in a time of need; we do it often when natural disaster hits. But if we did it with the intention to reverse the cause of illnesses instead of trying to find "cures," so many people would prevent or overcome their illnesses. We are obsessed with "cures" and Americans are always looking for a "quick fix." I'm here to tell you, there is no such thing as a "cure," and raising money for a "cure" is useless because it does NOT address a cause. Raising money for a "cure" merely promotes more scientists playing with chemistry in a lab so people can take a magical "pill" to "get better."

THE ROOT CAUSE

Through aggressive advertising, traditions, and propaganda, our minds are conditioned to become addicted and accustomed to a certain lifestyle, which includes unnatural foods, beverages, and desires. Over time, the lymphatic system gets congested, your pH level rises, and your organs and glands weaken from these harmful addictions that now manifest into illness. Once we get sick, we need to spend money to stay alive so we have more time to feed those addictions. All because we've been taught to think that this lifestyle is "living life to the fullest."

The aggressive advertising is meant to get children addicted so they become lifelong customers. Certainly Ronald McDonald, the Keebler Elf, and Tony the Tiger are not for me and you. Soda commercials often have kid themes, and the cereal aisle at the grocery store is nice and colorful. And how about when a kid's movie comes out, and they strike a deal with a fast food chain to cross promote it? And let's not forget the conditioning that goes on inside TV shows and movies. The Cookie Monster on *Sesame Street* is my personal all time favorite! "Mmmmmmm cooookie!"

SOCIAL MEDIA ASSIGNMENT:

What other negative programming and conditioning is out there directed at children? Think hard. Is it a TV commercial, a show, or a brand in general? I want to see your choices. Spread this awareness to your audience and inspire someone today.

TAGS: #StopBrainWashingKids #ThreeDLife #EatTheSunlight

And that's how the business of "consumables" works. They get you addicted and keep you coming back. All you have to do is watch television for three hours straight and write down all the commercials that sell products, which go into your bloodstream (food, beverages, gum, soaps, shampoos, make-up, lotions, over-the-counter medicines, and prescription pills). If you watch closely enough, you'll even see a commercial for junk food and medicine back to back. Don't blink!

Besides advertising, there are also traditions! Let's look at our precious holidays and see how they relate with food and beverages:

Holiday	Food & Beverages
New Year's	Alcohol, snack foods
Valentine's Day	Chocolate, candies, dining out
Easter / Passover	Flesh, starches, chocolate
Memorial Day	Cookouts
Mother's Day	Go out to dinner
Father's Day	Go out to dinner
Fourth of July	Cookouts
Labor Day	Cookouts
Halloween	Chocolate, candies
Thanksgiving	Flesh, starches, desserts
Christmas / Hanukkah	Flesh, starches, desserts

Perhaps no greater example of mind conditioning is better than that of Santa Claus. It's mind-blowing that we can actually manipulate and program a child's mind to believe that an overweight guy with a beard, who comes from the North Pole, flies around the world on a sleigh with reindeer. And if the child was good, this fictitious character will land on his or her roof, slide down the chimney, eat milk and cookies, and leave presents underneath a tree. The kids buy it hook, line, and sinker, and our culture helps as teachers, television, radio, and everyone in the "Christmas spirit" are all in on it. This is absolute proof that a child's mind is impressionable. So if that's the case, what do you think is happening to children's minds with the aggressive advertising, traditions, and propaganda that are consistently observed by their young minds with food and beverages?

It doesn't take long for those impressionable young minds to create strong memories, which are connected to their five senses. The "good feelings" they get through their senses manifest into addictions to certain foods, beverages, and desires. How many children do you know who won't throw a temper tantrum if they don't get their chicken nuggets, pizza, or ice cream?

Then, after many years of being a customer to those addictions and having poor genetics passed down from parents that went through the same cycle, malfunctions of the body will manifest. And as the malfunctions manifest through time, the kid, who is now an adult, will end up pouring money into the medical establishment to ease their physical suffering. And somewhere in this cycle, they may even have a child of their own they pass their poor genetics and habits to, which end up creating illnesses at even younger ages.

If that's not enough, we are also conditioned to be dramatic, angry, and opinionated from all the television, radio, and web video programing. From dramatic reality shows, to violent or ignorant web videos, to the five o'clock news, we are surrounded by conditioners that force stressors an untrained mind cannot handle correctly. This in turn creates poor health on the mind and body.

"Turn your radio and TV off and think for a second. Technology is a blessing, but it's also a weapon. A weapon of mass destruction giving global instructions, teaching us how to hate, but does it in a way that we love it."
- Germaine Williams

Therefore I tell you, mind conditioning is the root cause to past, current, and future illness. It leads to addictions, and addictions leads to malfunctions of the body; and that suffering leads to the medicine money pit!

I've found in my career that the most defensive people are the ones with illnesses. Telling them they can relieve or reverse their suffering is like telling them their kids are ugly. This is usually when we, the natural health practitioners, are referred to as "quacks" or "snake oil salesmen." I don't think we should blame the defensive person, for they were conditioned to think a certain way. They still believe in Santa Claus, and telling them that they've been deceived is hard for them to accept.

The Issue | You're Living in Unnatural Times

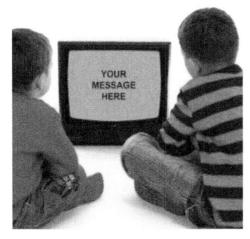

Harmful Foods & Products are Being Marketed to You

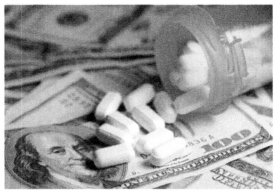

More Pills, More Money, More Side Effects, LESS Options

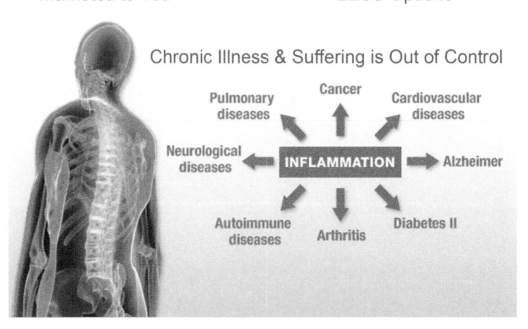

Chronic Illness & Suffering is Out of Control

Pulmonary diseases

Cancer

Cardiovascular diseases

Neurological diseases

INFLAMMATION

Alzheimer

Autoimmune diseases

Arthritis

Diabetes II

MEDICAL MONEY PIT

Can you believe the level of marketing they do with prescription drugs now? Colorful commercials with old people dancing or the "sick" person laughing and enjoying life, while the voice over person gives you details on the drug. They even make the "laundry list" of "precautions" sound happy and encouraging. Look deep and you will see that they're only promoting that you can live more comfortably with your illness by taking their product. The do not promote a "cure" or "reversal."

The IMS Institute for Healthcare Informatics reports that Americans spent $307 billion on prescription drugs in 2010. The ten drugs we spent the most amounts on were:

- Lipitor, a cholesterol-lowering statin drug—$7.2 billion
- Nexium, an antacid drug—$6.3 billion
- Plavix, a blood thinner—$6.1 billion
- Advair Diskus, an asthma inhaler—$4.7 billion
- Abilify, an antipsychotic drug—$4.6 billion
- Seroquel, an antipsychotic drug—$4.4 billion
- Singulair, an oral asthma drug—$4.1 billion
- Crestor, a cholesterol-lowering statin drug—$3.8 billion
- Actos, a diabetes drug—$3.5 billion
- Epogen, an injectable anemia drug—$3.3 billion

Treatment-based thinking makes a lot of money for the establishment. The way they do this is by first giving a group of symptoms a scary sounding name so it can be defined (diverticulitis, meningitis, endometriosis, etc). Once it has a scary name, not only can they now promote it as the monster that hides under your bed, but they can create a way to suppress the monster so it stays under the bed. And that suppression comes at a cost.

UNMASK THE MONSTER

I feel it's important that we start looking at the meanings behind the "scary" names. Let's look at some comparisons:

Fibromyalgia is a common syndrome where a person has long-term, body-wide pain and tenderness in the joints, muscles, tendons, and other soft tissues.

-VS-

Arthritis is inflammation of one or more joints. A joint is the area where two bones meet.

Now, let's do the skin…

Psoriasis is a common skin condition that causes skin redness and irritation.

-VS-

Eczema is a condition that causes the skin to become inflamed or irritated.

OK, now let's go to the stomach…

Irritable bowel syndrome (IBS) is a disorder that leads to abdominal pain and cramping, changes in bowel movements, and other unpleasant digestive symptoms.

-VS-

Colitis is swelling (inflammation) of the large intestine (colon).

My point is, illnesses come from the same causes no matter what scary name they give them! The medical establishment just needed names to make money off these "malfunctions" of the body. We can reverse the illness by reversing the cause. If you continue to follow the direction of your medic, he or she will "treat" your "disease" and suppress your "symptoms," which will keep you coming back for more of the "fix." And by doing this, you're still harboring the monster under your bed. This is clever mind conditioning, which makes billions of dollars.

Seems as though there's a lot of money to be made in the business of sickness, doesn't it? That's why the "establishment" will come and rip someone like me out of my house in the middle of the night. Because my colleagues and me don't need medicines and procedures to relieve people's pain. This ultimately takes money out of their pockets. It's like going to a corner in a tough neighborhood full of drug dealers, with a big sign that says "say no to drugs." Eventually, the drug dealers are going to come see you (that's street language).

The medical establishment basically own words like "disease," "cure," "treatment," and "diagnose," and they have designed it so anyone who isn't licensed to practice medicine cannot use these words freely without penalty. The system is also designed to go through your primary care physician. For only he or she can write you prescriptions or referrals to other specialty doctors. Your primary care physician holds a lot of your future in his or her hand. Now that's power.

But you can't get reasonable prices on prescriptions and medical appointments unless you pay for monthly memberships. That's right, they call this health insurance! I'll tell you, I pay about $150 a month, and I have no idea why. I propose that they create "emergency insurance" for folks like me. I have no need for medicine or a primary care physician unless I have an unfortunate accident.

And let me tell you from past experience, the ER is not cheap! The ER is where I need my coverage, as I am not getting much value for my membership. But, in America, I'm not allowed to go without a membership without penalty, am I?

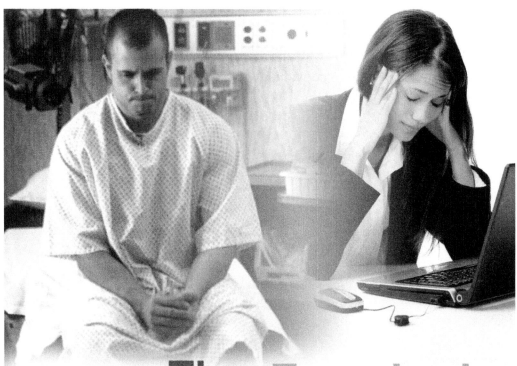

The Challenges | Everybody Has Them

Unsupported in Your Personal Development
Stress is Causing Exhaustion & Unhappiness
Hindered by a Condition or Illness
Unmotivated to Build New Habits
Overpowering Cravings or Addictions
Spending Unnecessary Money on Poor Health
Uneducated on Nutrition & Self-Care
Too Busy to Manage Your Own Well-Being

Do You Foresee Your Health Only Going Downhill?

WHO SAID?

Who said that cake goes with birthdays? Who said jewelry and fancy cars are status symbols? Who said that buttered popcorn goes with movie theaters? Who said women can be prettier with make-up? Who said our kids should leave Santa milk and cookies? Who said we should vote for a political party in November? Who said pizza, chicken wings, and beer goes with football? Who said you need chemo and radiation if you have cancer? Who said eggs, bacon, and sausage are breakfast foods? Who said alcohol goes with partying? Who said we should get yearly flu shots? Who said that coffee helps you wake up? Who said cigarettes are cool? Who said that overcooking flesh on grills goes with cookouts? Who said?

SOCIAL MEDIA ASSIGNMENT:

Join in on the "Who Said" game. What other stereotypes or mysteries can you think of that fit this topic? I want to see your choices. Spread this awareness to your audience.

TAGS: #WhoSaid #ThreeDLife #EatTheSunlight

Very truly, I say the establishment has built a system. A matrix. A cycle. A false image. And you are stuck inside the disillusioned design, which is meant for you to spend your hard-earned money on conditioned addictions which contribute to illnesses caused by those very desires. But as long as you are comforted with your pizza, burgers, fries, steak, soda, milk, cheese, cookies, cakes, candy, coffee, ice cream, tobacco, marijuana, alcohol, jewelry, video games, pornography, television, fancy cars, big houses, sports, blogs, Hollywood gossip, and of course, social media platforms to release your negativity…You think that you're "living life to the fullest."

My generation (I was born in 1979) is the fast/processed food era where we were brainwashed through new technologies that rose through the 80's, 90's, and 2000's. And with technology being created at a rapid rate, "they" can now condition our minds easier with more instant and effective marketing.

1980's—The rise of the microwave, diet sodas, and cable television

1990's—The rise of artificial foods like margarine, sour patches, and GMO's

2000's—The rise of the Internet, social networks, and Smartphones

TAKE A STAND

We spend the first half of our lives making ourselves sick, and the second half of our lives trying to make ourselves un-sick. It's a sad, harsh, and undeniable fact.

Maybe it's time to break free from living the establishment's way? Maybe it's time to step up and release ourselves from this programing and create a new lifestyle. A lifestyle that promotes a healthy body, a healthy mind, and a sick-free way of life. A lifestyle that will surely make us different than the people we work with, share public places with, and even live with, but yet makes us role models to others, as we become walking billboards for health and vitality. I think it's time to introduce the #ThreeDLife.

WHAT IS HEALTH AND VITALITY?

To a sports fan or commentator, "healthy" means being injury free. To a medical doctor, "healthy" means passing tests or having good blood work numbers. To a fitness buff, "healthy" means looking great and being strong. To an obese person, "healthy" means being skinny. To someone with a sickness, "healthy" means not having the sickness. The term "healthy" is all perspective.

It's hard to judge health because in order to do so, you must understand how the human body works. In other words, the twenty-three-year-old kid who consumes fast food, soda, and candy bars on a regular basis thinks he or she is healthy because he or she feels OK. But the harsh truth is, his or her lymph fluid is beginning to get congested, insides are becoming acidic, and certain organs and glands are beginning to weaken. Therefore, this young adult will become "unhealthy" by their standards any year now. It may take five years, it may take twenty years, but he or she will feel it eventually. Being "unhealthy" is a manifestation that happens over time. You are choosing to suffer later by making poor lifestyle decisions now.

In my opinion, health can't be defined until you hit forty years old. At forty, you can almost always feel the results of your lifestyle decisions you made as a teenager, young adult, and mature adult. If you can make it to forty and have never had an ailment or don't currently suffer physically or mentally, then you're probably "healthy." Notice I wrote "mentally" as well. It counts. Your thinking is just as important as your organs and glands.

The last time I checked, the average life expectancy in America is seventy-seven years old. It sounds good. But what they don't tell you is that in order to make it to that landmark age, you will have to live an artificial life that includes taking pills, supplements, and having procedures. Very rarely does a human make it to that age naturally. And that's because we live in unnatural times.

Allow me to use my family as an example. My grandfather died on the operating table during open-heart surgery at around fifty-years-old in 1972. His son, my father, survived on the operating table during open-heart surgery at around fifty-years-old in 1994. You see, they didn't have the technology in 1972 like they did in 1994; therefore, my father is still around as I write this book. So yes, he has an opportunity to make it to seventy-seven, but he has been suffering from poor health for a long time and will continue to suffer until he dies. He, like many American's are what I call "Darth Vader's;" people kept alive through technological means. That said, the life expectancy of America does not determine health. It just means technology is getting better.

I believe we should be living much longer, but these days, our lifestyles and genetic weaknesses take a toll and break us down in our sixties and seventies. I find it interesting that in the Bible, after the great flood, God declares man to live to one hundred and twenty years old. Is that age really possible?

"My spirit shall not strive with man forever, for he is indeed flesh, yet his days shall be one hundred and twenty years."

Here's a list of some recent people who lived that long:

Jeanne Calment	122 (died in 1997)
Shigechiyo Izumi	120 (died in 1986)
Sarah Knauss	119 (died in 1999)
Marie-Louise Meilleur	117 (died in 1998)
Lucy Hannah	117 (died in 1993)
Kamoto Hongo	116 (died in 2003)
Carrie C. White	116 (died in 1991)
Elizabeth Bolden	116 (died in 2006)
Tane Ikai	116 (died in 1995)
Maria Esther Heredia de Capovilla	116 (died in 2006)

I want you to understand that your lifestyle determines your health! What you eat, what you drink, the job you work, the way you think, the people you have relationships with, the way you handle stress, your hobbies, your interests—they all play a factor in being healthy. And they all lead to (or detract from) vitality.

Vitality is being strong and active. It's the energy, the zip, the motivation, the thrill, the passion you posses to live life to the fullest! It's the happiness you hold in your heart and drive you have to get up and go do things. Being in your sixties, taking a bunch of pills, walking gingerly, having a doctor for every body part, and spending most of your time watching television is not vitality.

A fantastic example of vitality is fitness pioneer Jack Lalanne. He opened what is considered the first health club in the 1930's and continued to be America's health guru for decades. He used to advocate a high meat and vegetable diet and later changed his view to fruits, vegetables, and moderate fish. But the two points he always advocated were fitness and staying away from artificially processed foods. You may remember him like I do, as being the "old guy" with tons of energy on the infomercials juicing fruits and vegetables. Jack Lalanne performed his daily exercise routine all the way up until the week he passed away, at the age of ninety-six. It's not his age that's impressive, it's how much vitality he possessed at his age that's impressive.

How will you feel at seventy? What kind of vitality will you posses? I've been known to tell my audience at my seminars that vitality is being seventy and doing push-ups! Having a quality of life that doesn't include unnecessary medicines, agonizing treatments, depression, resentment, anger, boredom, unhappiness, and fear is vitality. While your body will naturally break down as you get older, that doesn't mean you have to suffer like others do. The choice is up to you. Your life is your movie! You write it, direct it, and act in it.

I've created a yearly vitality test for you. It's a great measure as to how much vitality you have, and I think it's important to track it every year. Perhaps you can use New Year's or your birthday as a reminder to take your test. The goal should be to improve every year until you're in good standing.

SOCIAL MEDIA ASSIGNMENT:

If you're comfortable with posting it, I (along with the other people living the #ThreeDLife) would love to see your vitality score. Is there room for improvement? What was it last year? What do you want it to be next year?

TAGS: #VitalityTest #ThreeDLife #EatTheSunlight

The Yearly #ThreeDLife Vitality Test

Download a copy at KevinWReese.com/VitalityTest

Current Date: _____   *Current Age:* _____

How many times did you get sick this year?   _____

How many medications/medicines are you currently taking daily?   _____

What's your stress level on a scale of 1-10?   _____

How many hours of TV or video do you watch per week?   _____

Add up your numbers ----------------------------->   _____

Do you often feel physical aches or pains?   Yes _____ No _____

Do you often get constipated?   Yes _____ No _____

Do you often feel fatigued or sleepy?   Yes _____ No _____

Do you often have anxiety?   Yes _____ No _____

Do you argue often with family, friends, or a significant other?   Yes _____ No _____

Do you cry often or get depressed?   Yes _____ No _____

Are you addicted to something? (food, alcohol, sex, drugs)   Yes _____ No _____

Do you often get rashes or acne?   Yes _____ No _____

Do you often get heartburn or acid reflux?   Yes _____ No _____

Do you dislike your career or job?   Yes _____ No _____

Do you often get jealous?   Yes _____ No _____

Do you wish you went out and had fun more?   Yes _____ No _____

Do you wish you had an improved spiritual practice?   Yes _____ No _____

Add up your yeses ----------------------------->   _____

Perform as many sets in a row of 30 jumping jacks followed by 10 pushups.
Every set is worth 2 points. *Add up your fitness score* ----------------------->   _____

Total Score = Numbers + Yeses - Fitness ----------------------------->   _____

The Yearly #ThreeDLife Vitality Test

Download a copy at KevinWReese.com/VitalityTest

Great = *1-10*

Good =*10-20*

Poor = *20-30*

Horrible = *40*

#ThreeDLife
Success Stories

"For almost 20 years, I've had day-long migraines, as well as heavy bleeding and painful menstrual cycles related to fibroids. The Doctors were pushing me to get surgery, but I decided to learn the #ThreeDLife instead. Almost four months in, I didn't have any more cramping and my bleeding regulated. Before I knew it, my migraines were gone and my fibroids shrank! My Doctor said I no longer needed surgery."

- Keysha Rowe

WHAT IS THE #THREEDLIFE?

Through hours of training, working on my own health battles, and working with clients, I discovered that there needed to be a balance in one's life to achieve a certain level of health and vitality. You can't just be focused on your diet—it has to include the mind and it has to include cleansing your toxins and wastes. That's why I developed and coined the formula of DIET, DE-STRESS, DETOX.

You see, I found out that we can have the best diet in the world, but still be stressed out, and still get sick. I found that we could be stress-free, with a decent diet, but never clean our insides, and still get sick. One "D" will not work well without the other! This mind-blowing discovery led me to create this way of life and this amazing formula.

I've been using the #ThreeDLife on clients for a while, and the results are encouraging. Clients have paid thousands of dollars to do my program, but I felt the urgency to get this formula to as many people as possible, which is why I wrote this book. My hope is that I can properly translate my program and teachings into a word format so it can improve your life. In this book, I will attempt to explain the #ThreeDLife, and teach you how to apply it.

Before you continue, I want you to close this book and take a few minutes to focus on WHY you're reading my words in the first place. I often advise clients to write down their WHY and pin it to either their bathroom mirror or the ceiling above their bed. If you don't know your WHY, you will always TRY. And I don't want you to TRY, I want you to DO. But how can you DO, if you don't know WHY?

CHAPTER 2

INTRO TO THE HUMAN BODY

THE AMAZING MACHINE

In order to understand the #ThreeDLife, it's important to have a general understanding of the human body.

The human body is amazing! Organs, glands, and systems work without you telling them what to do. Your heart beats on its own. Your lungs breathe on their own. And your liver performs its hundreds of duties on its own. All living bodies operate and function as machines. What humans have over other animals is a very intelligent mind. This makes us superior as we can build houses, cities, cars, planes, and computers. But, this gift also makes us more ignorant too. We tend to overthink things and quickly lose touch with the laws of nature. This is our downfall.

The human body operates the same way today as it did centuries ago, and we must wrap our heads around that. Let's explore the human body briefly and see how it correlates to the #ThreeDLife.

CELLS & TISSUE

You're made up of tissue, which is comprised of trillions of cells. If I put your liver underneath a microscope, I would see cells. If I put your heart underneath a microscope, I would see cells. If I put your hair underneath a microscope, I would see cells. Each cell is alive. They are like little babies. They communicate, they cry, they eat, and they eliminate.

But what do they need to eat? Well, in order to make energy aka ATP (Adenosine Triphosphate), they need Carbon (C) and Oxygen (O2). Carbon is the root word for carbohydrate. Carbon is sugar. That's right, you need sugar to produce ATP! The simplest and most natural form of carbon we can eat is fruit (more on that later).

Let's talk about oxygen. Obviously, we are familiar with it because we breathe it everyday. But you can consume it too! There is oxygen in your water (H20), your fruits, and your vegetables. In fact, your greens contain chlorophyll, which helps circulate that oxygen to the cells. So every time you eat leafy greens like spinach, kale, or parsley, you are fueling your body with more oxygen to help feed those cells.

GENETICS

Inside the cell is what I call the "memory garden." In that "garden" is DNA, your genes, or your genetic constitution. All your information is there. What color your eyes are, the shape of your face, your features, etc. So if your mom had diabetes and your dad had arthritis, you're susceptible to chronic illness. Please understand, diabetes and arthritis are just words: The meanings behind the words will suggest that mom and dad are passing you a weakened pancreas, adrenals, and congested lymph system.

The good news is that you don't have to succumb to the genetic weaknesses you were given. Those seeds in the "garden" will only grow if you "water" them. You're going to "water" them by not getting enough proper carbon and oxygen. You will also "water" them by popping pills, smoking of any kind, being stressed, and of course, consuming way too much protein, artificial foods, refined sugar, and starches. Your fate is in your own hands. We have to stop blaming illness on genetics.

INTERVIEW WITH A SCIENTIST

In order to gain a better understanding of DNA and genetics, I interviewed my colleague and close friend, Coach Kevin Wright.

Coach Wright's background in biotechnology and immunology was refined over a decade-long career as a Research Scientist working toward the discovery of an AIDS Vaccine. With a high level understanding of biology, he brings a unique viewpoint on wellness and the healing of the human body. A graduate of Tufts University, The Institute for Integrative Nutrition, and the International School of Detoxification, we're happy to have him as a Chronic Illness Specialist on our team, as he inspires audiences to harness control over their health as well as their genetic destiny.

KWR: In your expert opinion, how would you describe what genetics is to someone who has no idea?

Coach Wright: Genetics was a fascinating study in college, certainly one of my favorite courses and highest marks. Beyond the detailed molecular mechanisms and patterns of inheritance, however, I've expanded my understanding of genetics to a level that is not only relevant to real world living but essential for empowering individual health journeys. It is the truth of our active participation in our own genetics. I call this 'the new genetics' because it is a level of understanding that you probably have never heard before.

The best and most simple way to describe the new genetics is as a symphony orchestra where genes are the various musical instruments, lifestyle habits are the musicians, and your health status is the musical sound of the symphony. So you, having control over your lifestyle habits, or musicians, play a vital role as conductor of your own great symphony of genetic expression.

Let's explore this further with some examples. You could have high quality instruments for your orchestra, but if they're being played by lazy and unrefined musicians, then the music won't sound so great. In other words, you can have great genes, but poor lifestyle habits will eventually yield a state of health that doesn't feel very good. On the flip side, you may have old beat up instruments, but your musicians are top class professionals. The sound of that symphony could be worthy of the stage at Carnegie Hall. That is to say, even if you have weaknesses in your genes, faithfully maintaining the lifestyle habits of the #ThreeDLife allows you to overcome those weaknesses and enjoy good health. Genetics is the interplay between your genes and your lifestyle and environment. It is the process of making your own symphony. You and you alone are the conductor.

KWR: Chronic illness and cancer is on the rise, especially in America. What role do you feel genetics play in this rise?

Coach Wright: Well, I don't believe it is encoded in our DNA; that's a false perception. The major blame is not on the instruments, it's on the musicians. The rise in chronic illness and cancer in this country is a direct result of modern trends in lifestyle and the environment. There's consistently more processed and manufactured foods, artificial preservatives and flavorings, toxic pesticides, herbicides, and fungicides, toxic cosmetics, isolated chemistry, microwaved food, air and water pollution, meat and dairy consumption, and stress. And at the same time, there's less exercise, living plant-based foods, personal responsibility, relaxation, deep breaths, love, and attention from doctors. Environment and lifestyle changes over the last 50 years have fueled the rise in chronic illness and cancer.

KWR: Do you feel it's possible for someone to change their genetic blueprint through lifestyle change?

Coach Wright: Well, you're not going to change your skin or hair color or the tone of your voice. Your particular set of instruments is what makes you, you. But certainly a natural #ThreeDlife can change the expression of your genes and reprogram your cells with new genetic memories. Consider it this way: If you fire your underperforming and neglectful musicians and hire brilliant new hard working musicians, they will not only make better music but will also take better care of their instruments, keeping them protected and polished. If your instruments are old and beat up, then over time, this new high level of care will actually improve the look and performance of your instruments. However, if your musicians are lazy and could care less, then over time, those instruments would deteriorate further and possibly start falling apart. Our lifestyle habits day in and day out affect the integrity of our genes. Genetic weaknesses can either be strengthened or worsened. We are in control of our own genetic destiny.

KWR: Do you think changing one's lifestyle and improving their genetics is necessary before having a child?

Coach Wright: Absolutely. I am very passionate about this message. I believe that every young couple should have access to this information—that babies do not come into this world with a clean slate. They are not born with brand new instruments. The condition of your instruments at the time of conception becomes the instruments that your child begins life with. This means that as a couple, you have the opportunity to polish up your instruments before handing them down to your next generation. You have the opportunity to choose a better set of musicians for the household where you'll raise your child. I cannot emphasize how critical this is for young couples and even singles who plan to have children one day. Think about this: All the damage done to your genes throughout your whole life will get passed down. Your 'now' point becomes your child's starting point. If your children start out with weaker genes, and they come into a toxic environment practicing the same damaging lifestyle, then they will develop chronic illness much sooner than it took you. We are seeing children today with serious illnesses! Kidney problems, cancer, asthma, diabetes…It's unreal.

They're coming into this world with serious weaknesses and stagnant lymphatic systems, and they are developing issues that we're used to seeing only in older adults. Before having children, you have the opportunity to do what you can to improve your child's health outcome. This is where the third 'D' in the #ThreeDLife is especially relevant. Get those instruments in the best shape possible before handing them down. And even if you already have children, getting them started on the #ThreeDLife as early as possible will have a long, lasting impression on their lives.

KWR: In your opinion, what plays a bigger factor in promoting chronic illness or cancer: genetics or lifestyle?

Coach Wright: The answer is simple—lifestyle. Chronic disease is not encoded in our genes—weaknesses are. Bad instruments don't make bad music; bad musicians do. It's possible to make beautiful music with bad instruments, but you may just have to work a little harder. One point I have to emphasize here is that most of us were unknowingly trained to be bad musicians; it's not our fault. But now that we know better, we have an opportunity to do better. Now that we understand the role we play in our own genetics, we can step up and conduct a new symphony. This is why it's so important to spread this message of the *Diet, De-stress, Detox* lifestyle. Everyone needs to know their own power.

KWR: If we as a people do not start improving our health and vitality, where do you see the future generations heading?

Coach Wright: Honestly, that future would be bleak. As I described earlier, each new generation doesn't start with a new clean slate. A baby is formed not out of thin air but from the existing cells of the mother and father. The condition of those cells at the time the baby is conceived become the starting condition of that new life in this world. We've been living wrong as a society for many generations, successively handing down older and worn out instruments. But the amount of damage that is being passed down within only the last two generations is frightening when you consider that this is the only time in history that we have entire generations coming up in a "McDonaldized" and "Monsanto'd" world. The level of genetic weakness is alarming. In the next two generations, we could see the collapse of human genetics, where the ability to conceive is lost and the survival rate of children plummets. We need to save our genetics! We have to do whatever we can to spread this #ThreeDLife awareness and reverse this trend.

KWR: What message do you want to convey to the readers?

Coach Wright: We are all endowed with beautiful sheet music, the encoded consciousness of Nature that makes us into living, breathing, thinking, loving beings. Our song is the human melody, a glorious expression of life. As a species, we were endowed with fine instruments and the responsibility to select quality musicians to play them. It's time that we come to realize our roles and responsibilities in our own human being-ness. We are the conductors of our own great symphony of genetic expression; we live and breathe and feel the experience of our own music, and our experience echoes into generations to come. Let's all go out and make beautiful music.

THE TWO FLUIDS

The trillions of cells that you're made up of need to be fed and cleaned just like a baby. That process happens with your two rivers of fluids that flow around your cells interstitially.

We're all familiar with blood. Blood has the large task of delivering the nutrients to these trillions of cells. This happens through four different ways:

1. What you swallow

2. What you inject

3. What you put on your skin

4. What you breathe

The hard truth about the four ways to feed the cells is that we can control three of the four. Certainly we can control what we swallow by eating and drinking the right foods and limiting or eliminating pills. We can control what we put on our skin with soaps, shampoos, lotions, and make-up. We can control going to get a flu shot or other vaccines. However, we generally can't control what we breathe.

If you're a tradesman of some sort and you're consistently in areas of possible asbestos or heavy metals, I personally would leave that environment alone. If you're addicted to smoking (of any kind), I personally would leave that alone as well (I quit Marijuana in 2008 and cigarettes in 2010). But we can't control the air outside. Our air is full of all sorts of pollutants from power plants, cars, and other machines. And with pollution and chemtrails all around us, this can be a problem.

The only remedy to combat the air is the third "D." Detox! Which we will talk about later.

Let's talk about cleaning the cells. Cells eliminate waste, just as a baby does. If you do not change a baby's diaper in ample time, what happens? Diaper rash, which leads to irritation and crying, right? And what you do not eliminate you accumulate!

We clean our cells with our other river of fluid in the body, which is called lymph. You may be familiar from popping a pimple or two in your day. That "puss" was just hardened stagnant lymph coming to the surface. Part of the lymphatic system, this fluid is our sanitation department. Its job is to remove your cellular wastes and toxins to the outside world. It does this through its drain, the kidneys.

LYMPH STAGNATION / CONGESTION

Imagine your lymphatic system as your city's sanitation department. Now imagine that department went on strike and the garbage man stopped coming to pick up the trash. What would happen to all your garbage in a few months? Would it start building up on your property? Would it start stinking? Would it attract bacteria, bugs, and rodents?

You want your lymph to be like a river, not a pond. You always want it to be moving. Nothing in life is good when stagnant. Once this lymph becomes stagnant, you're looking at congested pools of fluid, which harbor wastes, toxins, and acids. This is called toxemia.

The best analogy of toxemia is a pool. The reason we are able to swim in a pool is because it has a filter (kidneys). If you took the filter away, you would just have a big bucket of stagnant water. Is that something that sounds appealing to go swimming in? Now all the chemicals and wastes are going to simply start burning away at the bottom and sides of the pool. Eventually, malfunctions will occur, and the components that make up the pool will slowly break down.

When toxemia is pressing up against a gland or organ, it will eventually cause the tissue to weaken. After all, the gland is simply cells, right? When that internal gland or organ weakens, it will malfunction and cause a snowball effect of symptoms. Example: your adrenal glands. They do many things for your body, such as:

1. Sugar Metabolism (Type 2 Diabetes or Hypoglycemia)

2. Release Adrenaline (Anxiety)

3. Control Kidney Function (Blood Pressure, Bladder Issues)

4. Contribute to Lung Function (Asthma, COPD)

5. Contribute to Digestion Function (IBS, Constipation)

The point is, having weak adrenals will cause a slew of symptoms, which will send you to the MD. Your MD has a "treatment" for all five examples above, most of which include medications. But never will he or she help you achieve a remedy. Why? Because they were not trained to reverse the cause. Your MD will now treat the symptoms instead of the cause. The worst part is that most Americans don't know this and never fix the cause, which manifests into an artificial life full of suffering. Eventually, once you pass the chronic stage, you then experience the degeneration of the cells. You must move your lymph to bring your acids and waste to the outside world!

GOOD VS. EVIL

We are all familiar with the concept of good versus evil. We've experienced it in movies, television dramas, plays, the Bible, and our actual lives. Where there is a hero, there is a villain. And in health, it's the same thing. It's alkalinity versus acids. We can break this down in simpler terms by calling it cold versus hot.

Acids (hot) are the villains, and being corrosive, they burn, break down, and destroy our tissue (cells) over a period of time. Alkalinity (cold) puts that fire out and soothes the tissues. However, we need a small amount of acid to create a balance that gives your cells a proper environment to thrive. These are the two sides to chemistry, and it's detrimental that you have an understanding of this concept.

THE TWO SIDES TO CHEMISTRY

On a daily basis, you put either alkaline or acidic chemistry into your bloodstream. Everything from soaps, lotions, make-up, pills, gum, food, and beverages. It's all just simple chemistry. Which means they can be measured on the pH scale.

The pH scale is a measure of the hydrogen ion concentration. The scale goes from one to fourteen and 7.4 is considered perfect for the human body. You can get a pH test at your local natural health store.

When your body is in a state of too much acid, we call this acidosis. The medical establishment refers to it as inflammation. In my opinion, checking your pH is not a great measure. I say this because the human body will do tons of work to buffer the acid and bring it to a livable position. That's right, if your bloodstream becomes too acidic, you die. So the body works hard for you. Your body wants you to live. Of course, this happens at a great cost. Therefore, in my estimation, that makes the pH scale only useful for measuring the foods and beverages we consume.

Acids are basically protein foods, overcooked foods, smoke (of any kind), pills, and artificial foods. But no one acid former is consumed more consistently than protein. We're talking about flesh foods, dairy, eggs, some nuts, some seeds, beans, grains, and powders. I expand on this topic in my book *Protein Kills: Seven Reasons Why a High-Protein Diet Can Be Deadly*.

Let's explore acids some more. What do acids do? They burn! What happens when they burn? They inflame what ever it's touching! And sometimes, you don't even have to feel it. You can have silent inflammation too because it may not be touching any nerves. You won't even know it until pain or illness comes.

When's the last time you had a blue rash? When's the last time you had purple acne? Never! Because red is the color that is associated with fire. Those are acids seeping out of your skin via "the third kidney." When I take a client off of protein and artificial foods, they almost instantly break out in a rash. Why? Because their body was just given a chance to detox some acids while there are not as many coming in. Try it. Have a rash! It's on me!

When you consume acids, your pancreas doesn't have the proper enzymes to break it down for digestion. So, in order to break down acid, you need more acid! This is like the old saying "fight fire with fire." Can you imagine your house being on fire, and the fire department shows up and shoots fire on your house?

Your body has to produce hydrochloric, pepsin, and uric acids to break down the acid you're consuming. This creates an acidic experience inside your body. And if you do it on a consistent basis for many years, that acidic experience will manifest into an acidic environment. Once your body becomes an acidic environment, problems are going to arise.

One of many problems an acidic environment promotes is tumors and cysts. When you pour water onto dirt, it creates mud. Once you have mud, you can then form it into a ball, right? If you take that ball and leave it in the hot sun in the middle of July, what will happen? That wet mud ball will become hard as a rock because the heat dehydrated it and took the water out. That's how tumors and cysts happen. If your lymph fluid is stagnant, it creates a pocket of fluid (the mud ball), and if you have an acidic environment (hot sun in July), it's going to become hard as a rock.

Another big issue an acidic environment promotes is stones. Folks often wonder how the heck they got kidney or gallbladder stones, and the answer is simple. The acids coagulated together, and much like tumors and cysts, the acidic environment dehydrated them.

Some other problems from an acidic environment are gout, skin conditions, and cancer. I think it's safe to say when you're walking around with an acidic medium, you are just asking for trouble. You generally do not want to consume more than 20% of acid per day. If you smoke or take pills of any kind, that counts too.

PAIN

There are only two causes of physical pain:

1. Trauma

2. Acids

Practicing causality, if someone in pain comes to me for help, my first thought is, trauma or acids? With some people, such as athletes, it's both.

If you bang your knee, your knee will swell up with fluid. This trauma will cause your body to go through an immune response. What do you usually do in this situation? You put ice on it. What side of chemistry is the ice on? The alkaline side. It's a great way to put out the fire.

When acids inside of you burn, it causes inflammation. We've been conditioned to call it such words as arthritis, fibromyalgia, diverticulitis, IBS, and the list goes on. What do you usually do in this situation? You go to your MD and get pills. What side of chemistry are the pills on? The acid side. It's a great way to add fuel to the fire.

ARE YOU ON FIRE?

If your house is on fire, who do you call to help? The fire department. Well, so does your body. That's right, your body has its own personal fire department. If it didn't, most of you would be dead! So, if your insides are on fire (inflammation), your body has three separate fire departments it can call on:

1. Water

2. Cholesterol

3. Calcium

1. Edema (Water)

Just like that banged knee, your body will create water to put out a fire in your body. The medical establishment calls this edema. Have you ever known someone to say, "I shouldn't have eaten that. I'm so bloated now." If you know someone that has edema, you should instantly know, they're on fire! The example I like to use often in interviews and seminars is Bruce Lee.

In short, Mr. Lee died from cerebral edema at thirty-two. He was on painkillers (acids), ate a high protein diet (acids), reportedly smoked marijuana (acids and suppression of the adrenals), had lymph congestion in the head, which creates toxemia (wore glasses young), and one can assume, took some shots to the head during fights (trauma). All of these factors manifested into an accident waiting to happen. And it did when his friend gave him a pill to help his headache, and his brain filled up with too much water. His fire department had to create more water than it would have liked to. The acids won the war.

I use this Bruce Lee example often because it's proof of fitness not meaning true health. Mr. Lee was a fitness phenomenon but he was not healthy. If you want more information on this example, I have a video on my YouTube page where I go over how he died in better detail.

2. Cholesterol

Everyone knows someone with high cholesterol. Cholesterol plays an important role in the body. It contributes to the structure of cell walls. It makes up digestive acids in the intestine. It allows the body to produce vitamin D. And it enables the body to make certain hormones. But the big thing that no one talks about is it helps put out fires!

That's right, cholesterol is alkaline. The body will plaque it only if you are suffering from inflammation. Of course when cholesterol plaques it will lead to what the medical establishment calls "heart disease." But your body doesn't know that! Just like the Bruce Lee example, the body just knows it needs to put out your fire, or you will die.

3. Calcium

Haven't you ever met an older woman with a lack of calcium? Indeed, we need calcium for healthy bones, teeth, and nails. We need it to help with blood clotting and proper nervous system function. But guess what else it's needed for? You guessed it. To put out fires! Calcium is on the alkaline side of chemistry. In fact, when you have a tummy ache, what do most Americans do? They take an antacid. Check the ingredients and you will find calcium.

If you're on fire, your body is going to steal calcium from your connective tissues and bones to buffer the acids. This is going to lead to weak bones, poor teeth, brittle nails, and of course, potentially osteoporosis. This is robbing Peter to pay Paul.

YOUR EXITS

Earlier, I spoke of the entrances so that blood can "feed" the cells; now let me explain the exits, for it's the exits that you need for proper elimination. There are four main exits:

1. Kidneys/Bladder (Cellular Wastes)

2. Stomach/Bowels (Digestive Wastes)

3. Skin (Our Third Kidney)

4. Lungs (Release of Carbon Dioxide)

However, in a very congested body, there can be unnatural exits too. One that we are all familiar with is the mouth (vomiting). Others are our lymph nodes. It's been documented that women have shrunk and eliminated their breast tumors through their arm pits during natural healing modalities. This is because the job of the body is to eject the "impurity", and the armpit (lymph nodes) is the closest exit to the breast.

We need to eliminate. What doesn't get eliminated gets accumulated. If you ever go more than one day without having a bowel movement, I would highly recommend performing an enema (more on that later). You don't want your waste just sitting stagnant inside of you. Would you leave wastes sitting on your kitchen floor?

Speaking of getting rid of waste, the reason we nicknamed our skin the "third kidney" is because when our kidneys are not functioning properly, our waste tend to come out of our skin. So an indication of weak kidneys is chronic rashes or acne. Wherever that rash appears is also a sign of toxemia, as there is a pocket of lymph, which harbors acids that are coming out of the skin. And yep, it's not blue!

As for breathing, this is why we need good functioning lungs. Anyone with lung issues is going to accumulate even more acids, as they are not releasing enough carbon dioxide.

KIDNEYS

The kidneys are the filter or drain to your sanitation department (lymphatic system) and play a major role in detox. We need our kidneys for waste excretion, water level balancing, blood pressure regulation, red blood cell regulation, acid regulation, and more. If they are weak, we are going to end up in a war with acids. Just imagine driving on the highway, but the exits are blocked! There is no way out. Your waste will get backed up, just as the cars would.

As I said earlier, rash's are usually red. That's Acids. It's not an accident that most "gym rats" with their big muscles and protein shakes have poor skin. Many have acne broken out all over their shoulders and neck.

When protein structures get broken down, it creates waste, such as blood urea nitrogen (BUN). These wastes need to be removed. Then there is creatinine, which is a waste product of your muscles, and the more muscle you have, the more creatinine you have! If this waste builds up in the blood, it is a strong sign of weak kidneys. Anytime you have blood work done, your MD uses your BUN and creatinine levels as a measurement of kidney function.

After many years of abuse, your kidneys may start to leak protein into your urine. The medical establishment calls this proteinuria. We see this often with folks in their fifties, sixties and seventies. But these days, with the state of health going down the pooper, we are seeing it with people in their thirties and forties. Some symptoms might include foamy urine or swelling in your hands, feet, or face. You can have an UACR (Urine Albumin-to-Creatinine Ratio) test to find out your protein levels. If they come out high, you better lay off the protein…forever.

In detox, we want to get those kidneys opened up and filtering properly so that you can drain out your cellular wastes more effectively. Remember, each cell poops. A great way to see if your kidneys are filtering properly is to see if you have any whitish pulp in your urine. If you do, you're filtering, for these are wastes excreted from your lymphatic system and brought to the outside world through your kidneys. All you have to do is urinate in a jar first thing in the morning, and let the jar sit for the day. By night, the liquid will have settled and you can see what is floating in it. For someone that is filtering great, they will have whitish clouds of wastes that settle to the bottom. If you don't have any pulp, then you have work to do.

THE FOUR STEP PROCESS OF EATING & DRINKING

Knowing the process the body goes through when eating can be enlightening. But just know that what you eat becomes a part of you. You don't just eat a burger and fries and poop it out.

As you chew, you break the food up into mush that can be better broken down by the acids in your stomach. Once it leaves the stomach, it goes into the small intestine. It's in the small intestine where absorption takes place. Through the intestinal walls, your body takes the nutrients that it needs and wants. The nutrients then go into your bloodstream where they are circulated through the body to feed your trillions of cells. And finally, the leftovers that the body didn't use are sent to the large intestine, and are prepared to be eliminated. So your four step process is:

1. Digestion

2. Absorption

3. Utilization

4. Elimination

The two parts of the process that often contribute to poor health are digestion and absorption. If you have hardened mucioid matter built up in your walls, absorption will be hindered. This is how you have people that are skinny as a rail, but can never gain weight. I would bet they are experiencing malabsorption. These people usually end up with a chronic illness. If this is you, the detox section of this book will be useful to you to reverse your situation.

Utilization can manifest into poor health because if you're eating useless foods, you have nothing to utilize. Or if you're eating acidic foods, you're circulating acids that burn. In these cases, you are starving or burning your cells. Cells die in three ways:

1. Starvation

2. Acids

3. Trauma

Many people have problems with elimination as well. Again, what you don't eliminate, you accumulate. If you have problems with urination or bowel movements, you're in trouble. You are congested and need to detox yourself to restore your body back to removing your wastes frequently.

#ThreeDLife
Success Stories

"I started this program in a different place than I am now. Not only did I lose fifty pounds, but it's been an eye-opening and life changing experience. I thought the de-stress phase was going to be some different meditations, a yoga move here and an "omm" chant there, but I didn't expect it to be an introspective look at how we think and deal with things. There were issues I confronted that I had been dealing with since I was fourteen. It was an opportunity to let go of everything, and now when those topics come up in life, they roll off my back. The de-stress portion of this program gave me the opportunity to be the person I want to be. You know, people always tell you that you need to change, but no one ever gives you the "how-to" or the manual. This program gave me the manual. I'm very thankful that I have the tools and that understanding that I need to move forward with the #ThreeDLife. I'm only twenty-eight, and I have a lot of time to practice."

-Christina Outlaw

DUALITY

I had many chronic issues that developed through poor lifestyle choices. Here is a short list:

Varicose and spider veins on leg

Congested ear

Cyst removed from my left side

Chest pain

Headaches

You know what these "symptoms" all had in common? They were all on my left side! That's right, the veins were only on my left leg, the ear congestion was only in my left ear, the cyst was on my left side, my chest pains were in the heart area, and my headaches where around the left temple.

This was a clear indication that I had lymphatic stagnation/congestion on the left side of my body. When I learned this, it set me free of my worries, because I now knew how to work toward a remedy.

You see, we are split in half. We have two legs, arms, nostrils, kidneys, testicles/ovaries, eyes, ears, adrenals, and the list goes on. This is why, when you get your blood pressure taken, it would be good to get done on both sides.

THE HUMAN DIGESTIVE SYSTEM

In order to fully understand what you should be eating, one should understand what kind of digestive system you have. Let's look at animals.

Are you a carnivore? No. If you were, you could chase down a deer, bring it down with your teeth, and eat it on the spot with no fire. If you are able to do that, then we need to get you in the next vampire movie! The most famous carnivore is a cat. Not just lions and tigers, but your pet cat. Your cat can catch a mouse or a small rodent and actually consume and digest the bones. That's because its GI tract is short and provides enough acid to do such. You can't do that. You have to cheat and use fire to make flesh consumable for you. And just because you can eat flesh doesn't mean you're supposed to. We're not supposed to kill and steal, but we still do, right?

Are you an herbivore? No. If you were, you could go outside right now and eat the grass or the bushes. You would throw-up because you cannot properly digest it. It's too coarse and you do not have the proper molars or a long enough GI tract to process those type of greens. This is why we juice wheatgrass, because we can't eat wheatgrass! Plus, herbivores have multiple stomachs. Horses, elephants, cows, giraffes, etc. all have multiple stomachs that are designed to break down these thick greens. You can see evidence of improper digestion when you eat too many leafy greens, like spinach or kale. That's right, look down, and you will see green poop (don't act like you've never looked!).

So, if you're not a carnivore or an herbivore, you are definitely not an omnivore, which can eat flesh and grass. Those are bears, dogs, chicken, and pigs. OK, then what kind of digestive system do you have?

Well, name another animal that can peel an orange or a banana? Name another animal that walks upright on two legs? Name another animal that has a tailbone verses a tail? Name another animal with opposable thumbs? Name another animal that makes simple tools in the wild? Name another animal that can give you the middle finger…?

It just so happens that our digestive system is almost identical to apes!

Carnivores

Who:
-Cats, lions, tigers, wolves, etc.

Diet:
-Mostly flesh, moderate greens

Digestive System:
-The liver is 50 percent larger than humans and has five distinct chambers with heavy bile flow with gastric juices.
-They have no salivary glands. Their tongues are rough for pulling and tearing.
-Their small intestines are smooth and short.
-Their colons are non-sacculated and have minimal ability for absorption.
-Their GI tracts are three times the length of the spine.

Extremities
-Include sharp claws, and they walk on all four legs.

Integumentary System
-100 percent covered with hair, and they use their tongues and padded footpads as their sweat glands.

Teeth
-Incisors in front, molars behind with large canine teeth for ripping. Their jaws are unidirectional, up and down only.

Tail?
-Yes

Kidneys
-Meant to handle and eliminate acids.

Herbivores

Who:
-Horses, deer, elephants, cows, sheep, etc.

Diet:
-Mostly greens, moderate roots and barks

Digestive System:
-Their salivary glands are meant for alkaline digestion as they are oblong, ringed, and do not handle acids well.
-Their small intestines are long and sacculated for extensive absorption.
-Their liver is similar to a human's.
-Their tongues are moderately rough.
-Their colons are also long and sacculated for extensive absorption.
-Their GI tracts are thirty times the length of the spine.

Extremities
-They have hoofs and walk on all four legs.

Integumentary System
-They have pores with extensive hair covering entire body. Their sweat glands include millions of perspiration ducts.

Teeth
-They have twenty-four molars, five on each side of the each jaw and eight incisors for cutting. Their jaws are multi-directional, up and down, side to side, forward and backward, creating a grinding effect.

Tail?
-Yes

Kidneys
-Meant to handle and eliminate alkalinity, not acids.

Omnivores

Who:
-Bears, pigs, birds, dogs, etc.

Diet:
-Combination of flesh, greens, fruits, roots and barks.

Digestive System:
-Their salivary glands are underactive.
-Their stomachs have moderate gastric acids (HCL & Pepsin).
-Their small intestines are somewhat sacculated, which accounts for their ability to eat greens.
-Their livers are complex and larger proportionality than humans.
-Their colons are shorter than humans, with minimal absorption.
-Their GI tracts are ten times the length of the spine.
-Their tongues are moderate to rough.

Extremities
-They have hoofs, claws, and paws and walk on four legs (except for birds).

Integumentary System
-They have smooth, oily hair or feathers. Their sweat glands are minimal and are only around the snout (pigs) and footpads (dogs).

Teeth
-They have tusk-like canine teeth or beaks and their jaws are multi-directional.

Tail?
Yes

Kidneys
-Meant to handle and eliminate both alkalinity and acids.

Frugivores

Who:
-Primates and Humans

Diet:
-Mostly fruits, moderate greens, root vegetables, nuts, seeds, herbs, sprouts.

Digestive System:
-Their salivary glands are alkaline.
-Their stomachs are oblong with two compartments.
-Their stomachs have moderate gastric acids (HCL & Pepsin).
-Their small intestines are sacculated for extensive absorption.
-Their livers are simple and average size, not large and complex like carnivores.
-Their colons are sacculated for extensive absorption.
-Their GI tracts are twelve times the length of the spine.
-Their tongues are smooth and used mainly as a shovel.

Extremities
-They have hands with four fingers and a thumb meant for picking, peeling, scraping, and tearing. They have feet with toes. And they walk upright on two legs.

Integumentary System
-They have pores with minimal hair, and sweat glands that include millions of perspiration ducts.

Teeth
-They have thirty-two teeth. Four incisors for cutting, two cuspids that are pointed, four small molars (bicuspids), and six molars (no long canine or tusk type teeth).

Tail?
-No (some small primates, but not apes).

Kidneys
-Meant to handle and eliminate alkalinity not acids.

MACHINE RECAP

Through my education and experiences, I like to visualize the human body as a tube and tank machine with an electrical system that is made up of trillions of cells and two major fluids all designed to create and react to chemistry.

When you look at your body as such, it's easier to understand when pain or discomfort happens. Tubes and tanks can have blockages or tighten, electricity can short circuit or weaken, cells can weaken and eventually degenerate, and fluids can stagnate or carry harmful chemistry which creates negative reactions.

We know that machines can malfunction, but we also know that machines can be fixed. Your body is a living organism that knows what it's doing. We know this by having a history of broken bones and cuts on our flesh. When a medic places your bones back together, the break eventually heals and the bones mend. When you have a cut on your skin, it also heals back together as your machine creates a scab. What makes you think your insides can't do the same?

CHAPTER 3
DIET

WHAT DOES DIET REALLY MEAN?

When I say diet, I don't mean "going on a diet" or "dieting." It just simply means what foods and beverages you consume on a daily basis. If I ask you what your diet looks like, you should be able to tell me what an average day consists of from breakfast to bedtime.

In the 90's, the soda companies hurt the word diet by coming out with diet soda. Why couldn't they have just named it sugar free? Why the word diet? How many times have you heard a woman say, "I have a wedding coming up. I need to go on a diet." Or, "I feel horrible. I'm off my diet." Unfortunately, our society has ruined the word diet. So many diets have come out over the decades, and these have caused people to become confused. The problem is that most diets have to do with weight loss.

WEIGHT DOESN'T MATTER

Weight loss is a scam. We constantly see advertising for burgers, pizza, and ice cream, yet we also constantly see celebrities showing their abs. So now we have a ton of people overweight, feeling miserable, and wishing they looked like a celebrity. You see, we're conditioned to care about our looks! It's a vulnerability, and there's a lot of money to be made in human vulnerability. This is why infomercials thrive on late night television. They appeal to the vulnerable person.

How many pills and powders are on the market that promote weight loss? How many guest appearances on TV shows are there that highlight the newest and best way to lose weight? How many before and after pictures must you see before you crack and spend money on another weight loss diet or exercise machine? Weight loss is a big business!

I don't think that weight matters. Chronic illness does not discriminate. Acidosis does not discriminate. Physical pain and even death do not discriminate. Haven't you ever met someone with lupus, arthritis, fibromyalgia, migraines, or diverticulitis that are not overweight? Haven't you ever known someone to live into their nineties who's fat? Haven't you ever heard of a professional athlete dying young from a heart attack or from cancer?

Earlier, I gave the example of Bruce Lee , but certainly, he is not the only one. Many athletes have died young. Lou Gehrig died at the age of thirty-seven from ALS. Ernie Davis died at twenty-three from leukemia. Reggie White suffered from pulmonary sarcoidosis and sleep apnea and died at the age of forty-three from cardiac arrhythmia. Hank Gathers, twenty-three, and Reggie Lewis, twenty-seven, both died from hypertrophic cardiomyopathy. Darryl Kile died at thirty-three from coronary disease. Manute Bol died at forty-seven from kidney failure. Dennis Johnson died at fifty-two from a heart attack. Pete Maravich died at forty from a heart attack. And the Ultimate Warrior just recently died at fifty-four from a heart attack.

How about chronic illness? Dwayne Wade suffers from migraines. Venus Williams with Sjogren's syndrome. Jay Cutler with type 1 diabetes. Kevin Dineen with crohn's disease. Tim Raines with lupus. Shaquille O'neal with arthritis.

So, everyone I just named is or was a professional "in-shape" athlete. So why do they suffer or die? Do you still think weight matters? Do you still think being in shape matters? Are you ready for true health? Are you ready for vitality?

NUTRITION

Can you imagine a lion not eating the freshly killed zebra because of the grams of fat? Can you imagine a cow eating grass because it heard that the chlorophyll is good for them? Can you imagine a gorilla eating an orange because it wants vitamin C? I certainly can't imagine these things because they're more than likely not true! Animals use instinct. They don't know the specifics of the nutrients or value of their food. But they know what they're supposed to eat, and they don't get chronic illnesses.

You have to wonder why the "establishment" came up with food labels. In my view, it was to put value on certain categories like calories, fat, protein, and cholesterol in order to sell other items. Let's use fat as an example: when the media started promoting that fat was "bad", the food companies capitalized by creating artificial "fat-free" products. Now, they can throw a "fat-free" label on it and mention it in the television commercial. You see this exploitation with protein often, and "gluten-free" is becoming trendy now as well.

Some health and fitness gurus promote "superfoods" or "nutrient dense" foods. I feel that it's just another way to sound like an expert to sell their program, book, or idea. Every human on earth knows that fruits and vegetables are good. All fruits and vegetables are super foods and are nutrient dense as they're full of vitamins, minerals, and phytochemicals.

Is it that big of a deal that one knows what vitamins, minerals, and phytochemicals are in kale, broccoli, and apples? Before you call me a hypocrite, yes, I promote the value of certain plant foods with my "Sunlight Rap" series on my YouTube channel. But it's a clever and fun way to get folks excited, especially kids. On the practitioner side, I like to know what certain foods contain, but that is for protocol purposes. For example, when a client comes to me with say, asthma, I know what foods help with the lungs and adrenals. Using foods to heal is protocol. Your normal diet is not protocol; it's maintenance.

MACRONUTRIENTS

The three macronutrients are:

1. Carbohydrates

2. Protein

3. Fat

It's generally taught that the human diet should be 70 percent carbs, 15 percent fats and 15 percent protein. I feel this is nutrition mumbo jumbo.

Of course carbs should be a majority of our diet so you can get the carbon you need, but the problem is no one knows what carbs are! We have to start looking at the meaning of words and stop concentrating on the titles themselves. What kind of fats? What kinds of protein? When you live the #ThreeDLife and you #EatTheSunlight, it's specific. We need to be specific! It's like, OK, you live in a house. How big is the house? Where is the house located? How many floors are in the house? Do you have a basement? What's the condition of the roof on this house? Specific please.

SIMPLE VS. COMPLEX

Another concept in our diets that's important to know is simple versus complex. Complex means the food is a long chain of some sort of element. Hence, we call this a structure. But the truth of this is the body does NOT use structures. The body must break down structures into its simplest form in order to find it useful. In doing so, the body has to put in extra work.

The simpler you eat, the more efficiently the human body will function. Eating a simple diet will provide you a true energy that promotes vitality.

Knowing this information, can you imagine how something such as a bacon, egg, and cheese on a bagel bogs you down? The body has to put in all that work for a simple five minutes of satisfaction. My goodness. You just won't realize it until you #EatTheSunlight for a month or two, and you feel like you can run marathons and climb mountains.

Complex Foods

CARBS - Polysaccharides (Potatoes, Grains, Pastas)

PROTEIN - Complete (flesh, dairy, eggs, powders)

FAT - Polyunsaturated / Saturated (flesh, dairy, eggs)

Simple Foods

CARBS - Monosaccharaides (fruits & greens)

PROTEIN - Amino Acids (fruits & greens)

FAT - Monounsaturated (nuts & seeds)

FRUIT IS YOUR SUPERHERO

As we discovered earlier, our digestive systems and overall bodies are most similar to apes. That makes us, like apes, a frugivore! And a frugivore's GI tract is designed for fruit!

The strongest ape is the gorilla, which eats a 90 percent fruit diet, yet is one of the strongest animals walking this earth. However, if you want to get specific, scientists have estimated over the years that we share 99 percent of our DNA with another ape, the chimpanzee. In fact, humans are so similar to chimps, that the asymmetry of a chimpanzee's brain and its hand preference (left or right) is parallel to ours. Is there another wild animal that can be left-handed? Other animals don't even have hands—they have paws!

A chimps diet is 50 percent fruit, supplemented with greens, nuts, seeds, bark, blossoms, and insects. Very rarely will an ape hunt other mammals and eat their flesh, and when they do, it's usually for dominance reasons.

If you gave an orange to your dog, it would think it's a ball. Can you picture a lion trying to open a mango? What would a rabbit do with a watermelon? Certain animals are meant to eat certain foods, and it just so happens that you and apes are meant to pick, peel, scrape out seeds, and perfectly chew and digest fruit.

Yes, I know what some of you are thinking. "What about the sugar?" I had a client the other night tell me that her co-workers were aggressively informing her that she shouldn't be eating that much watermelon, and it was just pure water and sugar. This is pure ignorance brought about by programming from the "establishment." If it was true, I would have chronic illnesses and more importantly, so would the primates. I'm here to tell you, fructose is a natural simple sugar. It's a monosaccharide that is metabolized easier than any other food we could put in our mouths. Complex carbs (starches, such as bread, potatoes, pastas, and flours) are long chains of carbon that leave behind "sugar leftovers" because the body can't metabolize these structures properly. This brings forth fungus, belly fat, and can cause your sugar levels to spike. So it's not how much sugar is in a food—it's what *kind* of sugar is in a food!

When I teach children, I refer to the fructose in fruit as "Sunlight Sugar." It's magical and incomparable to table sugar or the refined sugar put in cookies and candy. It's the best kind of simple carbon you can get. And remember, you need carbon and oxygen to create vital energy. What other foods are better? Grains? Beans? Pastas? Breads? Flesh? Dairy? You know what these foods have in common? They all can't be consumed in their natural state! You have to soak them, or boil them, or pasteurize them, or cook them, or add ingredients. These denatured foods can manifest into poor health as they cause immune responses in the body. Why would the human body react that way toward these foods? Because they're recognized as foreign. It's like breaking into a department store and the alarm is going off! Intruder! Intruder! Intruder!

Fruit is special. Think about how many flavors there are. Is there another food on this planet that has the variety of tastes that fruit does? Is there another food that even tastes good in its natural state at all? Even the "establishment" knows this; that's why they use fruit flavors for your fake, destructive, artificial foods, like candy, gum, and ice cream. The same person who criticized my client for eating too much watermelon probably sucks on watermelon-flavored candy, drinks cherry soda, or feeds their kids orange-flavored popsicles.

And if that's not enough reason, isn't fruit one of the only natural foods that you don't have to refrigerate (nuts and seeds too)? They take a long time to start decomposing, don't they? The only fruits I put in the fridge are berries (grapes included) because they tend to ripen fast. But my apples, oranges, melons, mangoes, pears, pineapples, and peppers all stay in a big old basket I bought. You can't leave kale or spinach un-bagged in a basket, can you? You can't leave flesh or dairy out on the counter, can you? No! They all oxidize and then go bad.

As you start to incorporate more fruit into your daily diet, you may get slight stomachaches, rumbling, or acidity. In fact, I had a client just the other day say that her stomach was rumbling real loud at her job from eating too much fruit. She was discouraged and embarrassed. The first reaction is the blame the fruit! So I asked what she ate the day before. Turns out it was junk! The reason for the tummy noise was because fruit is astringent, meaning it's a cleaner. So, it's cleaning up your gut and mixing with the "junk" that is already leftover in your tummy. So let's not blame the fruit for doing it's job. If you ate a high-fruit diet, you wouldn't get the stomachaches, rumbling, or acidity because you would be clean. Remember, this food stuff is all chemistry!

Diet

Fruit is always the answer to the human body, and I'll tell you why:

1. Juicy fruits such as grapes, berries, and melons move lymph.

2. Fruit gives natural energy with no spikes and crashes like "sweets."

3. The fructose in fruit needs no insulin. It diffuses through the cells.

4. A piece of fruit digests in about an hour.

5. Fruit is full of vitamins and minerals.

6. Fruit is full of fiber.

7. Fruits are on the alkaline side of chemistry.

8. Fruit helps the nervous system, giving you clarity and focus.

9. There are so many kinds, with so many flavors.

10. Most nuts and seeds come from fruits, which makes it a complete food group.

11. Fruit is astringent and cleans and sweeps out toxins and wastes.

12. Fruits don't need to be denatured, so you can eat them raw. This makes fruit real fast food.

I recommend you always eat one fruit at a time, which is called a mono meal. But I like to refer to it as a #MonkeyMeal. It's a fun and easy way for clients to remember the rule while harnessing the ultimate power of your "superhero" (fruit). The reason for the mono meal is for digestive purposes (I'll explain this later) as you create a natural alignment within your GI tract.

So, if you're going to eat oranges, grab five of them and chow down! If you're going to eat a melon, split it open, grab a spoon, and dig in. If you're going to eat apples, maybe cut up three to five of them, and you can even sprinkle some cinnamon on them for an "raw" apple pie. Be a monkey! Let your superhero take care of you!

SOCIAL MEDIA ASSIGNMENT:

Post your monkey meals. Spread this awareness to your audience and inspire someone today. I want to see all different types of fruits. Flash your colors!

TAGS: #MonkeyMeal #ThreeDLife #EatTheSunlight #Superhero

MONKEY MEAL
aka The Mono Fruit Meal

PICK A SWEET FRUIT - APPLES, ORANGES, GRAPES, ETC
EAT AS MUCH OF THAT FRUIT AS YOU CAN FOR A MEAL

WHY?

- FRUIT PROVIDES ENERGY BY BEING THE ULTIMATE CONSUMABLE SIMPLE CARBON ON EARTH
- FRUIT IS AN ASTRINGENT, SO IT PROMOTES CLEANING
- FRUIT DIGESTS EASIER AND FASTER IN THE HUMAN BODY THAN ANY OTHER FOOD
- FRUIT IS FULL OF VITAMINS
- FRUIT MOVES LYMPH
- CONSUMING ONE KIND OF FRUIT AT A TIME MAKES IT EASIER TO DIGEST. SO YOU'RE SAVING YOUR BODY MASSIVE AMOUNTS OF ENERGY
- YOUR DIGESTIVE SYSTEM IS ALMOST IDENTICAL TO PRIMATES

SUNLIGHT SUGGESTION 1:
Have your Monkey Meal midday or afternoon so you can use the energy

SUNLIGHT SUGGESTION 2:
Try Peppers and Cucumbers too, they're also Fruit

SUNLIGHT SUGGESTION 3:
For the first Month or so, you will feel hungry and unsatisfied. But your body will adjust. Plus, you can eat as much as you need or want

www.EATTHESUNLIGHT.com

Fruit is always best in season. It will taste better and the nutritional value will be most vibrant. That's not to say you can't eat fruit out of season. But here is a general list.

Apples	September & October
Apricots	July
Avocado	May - November
Banana	January & December
Bell Peppers	September & October
Blackberry	July & August
Blueberry	July & August
Cherries	June
Cucumbers	July & August
Dates	September & October
Figs	July - September
Grapes	July -September
Kiwi	December - February
Mango	May - August
Melon	June - August
Nectarines	June - September
Oranges	December - April
Peaches	July - September
Pears	August & September
Pineapples	June - August
Plums	August & September
Pomegranates	October - November
Raspberries	July & August
Strawberries	April - May
Squash	July & August
Tomatoes	July - October
Zucchini	July & August

SUGAR

It's important to understand it's not how much sugar you consume—it's what kind of sugar you consume! An apple is sugar. A cookie is sugar. The white powder you put in your coffee is sugar. A piece of bread is sugar. Candy is sugar. Pasta is sugar. Are they all equal? Far from it.

There are short chains of carbon (monosaccharaides) and long chains of carbon (polysaccharides). The most famous long chain of carbon is what we call starches. However, most people refer to them as "carbs." These are breads, potatoes, grains, pasta, etc., and they are complex whereas fruit is simple.

The sugar in "sweets" such as candy or cookies is called sucrose or table sugar. This powder is taken from a sugar cane and is usually refined or processed. This type of sugar is denatured and highly addictive. It is said to be more addictive than heroin. Haven't you ever noticed little kids craving sweets? And adults for that matter? Look how many people are addicted to soda! I've had clients that have trouble getting off of chocolate. This kind of sugar is a drug.

I realize that there are some diabetics reading this book right now, and they are scratching their heads about eating fruit. I know this because they do it at my live seminars! Yes, you can and should be eating fruit! It's the simplest carbon on earth, and is what your cells need. And yes, it can contribute to some blood sugar spikes in the beginning as your body adjusts. But there are other factors too. For example, your adrenal glands put out a hormone called cortisol, which creates fluctuations in blood sugar. Your adrenal glands are directly connected to stress. That said, stress spikes your blood sugar too, and I don't see many people avoiding that!

Most fruit has a low glycemic load (GL). The GL of food is a number that estimates how much the food will raise a person's blood sugar after consuming. GL is based on the glycemic index and is defined as the fraction of available carbohydrate in the food multiplied by the food's GI. A starch has a high GL and will not only spike your blood sugar, but will cause that blood sugar to crash. This is when diabetics get sleepy and usually get knocked out cold. Fruit doesn't crash because it's a simple sugar and there aren't "leftovers," like after eating a starch structure.

I've had diabetics eat fruit and then hours later, they're eating a starch because their blood sugar level is too low! They can't believe it. It's at that point that they realize they were told not to eat fruit out of ignorance.

STARCHES

Starches (or polysaccharides) are long chains of carbon. These structures are hard to break down by the body, and the leftover remains promote candida, parasites in the gut, and belly fat. Starches are gluey and don't travel through our GI tract very well, which brings forth hardened mucoid plaque. And if that isn't enough, starches are also mucus-forming, which contributes greatly to stagnating our lymph fluid. This stagnation can lead to toxemia.

Folks often binge on starches as they never seem to fill us up. What they do not understand is the effect these complex foods actually have on your body. Your body must go through a tremendous amount of work to break down long chains of carbon because they're consumed as structures. However, a starch is still better than protein because there is no valuable carbon in protein. The cells want simple glucose and fructose (fruits and most vegetables) so it can make ATP.

Many people often limit these "carbs" to avoid getting fat. The high-protein, low "carb" diet is very dangerous because you are starving your cells of enough carbon. I go over this in depth in my book *Protein Kills: Seven Reasons Why a High-Protein Diet Can Be Deadly.*

America is going through a gluten phase right now. Everywhere you look there is something marketed as "gluten-free," as they try to make a buck off of folks who are gluten sensitive. Gluten is mostly in starches, but even if gluten isn't in a starch food, it still doesn't make the starch food good for the human body. You will notice that many people that have sinus "allergies" are big starch eaters.

Pastas, breads, and grains can lead to many poor health conditions. I know what some of you are thinking: "But what about Chinese people? They eat tons of rice and are skinny!" Well, as I mentioned earlier, weight doesn't matter. Many skinny people are skinny because they have malabsorption issues from mucoid matter hardened and pressed against their GI tract walls. If one has malabsorption, then they will NOT gain weight! Starch is a major contributor to creating mucoid matter.

#EatTheSunlight foods can be grouped as fruits, vegetables, nuts, seeds, herbs, and sprouts (more on this later). The only starch that falls under this category is potatoes. Potatoes are a root vegetable and can be eaten without being denatured (if you wanted to). Pastas, breads, and grains must be denatured to be consumed by a human. This causes an immune response.

Potatoes contain some really great nutrition, including B vitamins and vitamin D. They go great with leafy greens, marinated vegetable dishes, and make a good mono meal. That said, they do spike your blood sugar, and at the end of they day, they are still a starch. You can eat them in the #ThreeDLife, but I recommend that you heed the following:

1. Don't fry your potatoes because then they becomes toxic.

2. Eat potatoes no more than once or twice per week to limit candida and belly fat.

3. Never mix with protein (more on this later).

It's important to note: Corn is the only grain-starch that doesn't need to be denatured to consume. You don't have to cook corn. Corn is great for making soups, dressings, or eating as a mono meal. So technically, corn can be considered sunlight too. But like potatoes, corn should be eaten in moderation, as it's still a starch!

While we're at it, what other starches besides corn and potatoes have any natural taste? Have you ever been excited to eat plain rice or bread? Or do you need other "foods" to put on them to give them flavor?

If you look at the original food pyramid, in the 1990's, the US government published the pyramid with starches on the bottom, making it America's number one food group. No wonder Americans are full of chronic illnesses. Their lymph fluid isn't moving!

#ThreeDLife
Success Stories

"I think I've changed tremendously. I'm calmer and more focused. I used to have stress about what others thought about me and if I was a good enough mother. And now what others think doesn't define me. The diet has been life changing. If you told me I would be satisfied eating fruits and vegetables with low protein and no bread, I would tell you there is no way that would happen. Now, I feel like crap if I don't Eat the Sunlight. I know it's right for me. And I can tell others think it's right for me because of the compliments. And it's not hard. I always thought this diet would be hard. So overall, I've changed my mindset. It's about me and my health and making my family healthy and not what others think of me."

-Jen O'Keefe

VEGETABLES

If fruits are your superhero, greens are their sidekick!

Notice I'm using the term "greens." That's because "vegetable" has too big of a meaning. Again, we have to start looking at the meanings *behind* the words. Potatoes are vegetables, so technically, you can go chow down on French fries and get your "daily serving" of veggies. Add some ketchup while you're at it, and you will meet the USDA's food requirements!

Veggies, much like the foods I listed above, don't generally taste good in their natural state. In order to make them taste good, you have to use marinades, spices, and cook them. It's important to understand that squash, peppers, cucumbers, and tomatoes are technically fruits. They have seeds. Fruit is birthed off of a bush or tree; vegetables are the plant, as they grow directly from the dirt.

That said, can you name another vegetable, besides maybe carrots and beets, that taste good in nature? This is why the salad is so important! A salad provides an opportunity to get a ton of quality foods and make them taste good with spices and dressings, all while still keeping it raw.

As you may have heard from the #EatTheSunlight kid song or at my seminars, I do use the word vegetable when teaching a wide audience. But truly, it's the greens that matter. Greens are the second most important food for the human body. They essentially consist of everything we were programmed to think flesh provides: magnesium, iron, calcium, amino acids, protein, and more.

But most importantly, they contain chlorophyll, which is how they got their green color. Through a process brought on by the sunlight called photosynthesis, these greens (especially leafy greens) help circulate your oxygen. And I remind you again that your cells need carbon and oxygen to create vital energy.

I like using the term "greens" because it makes it easy to remember. Anything green is a must have! It can be a fruit, herb, leaf, or a stem. Here are some quality greens:

Celery

Spinach

Broccoli

Kale

Parsley

Romaine

Dill

Basil

Chard

Dandelion Greens

But, as I taught you earlier, you cannot digest leafy greens as well as fruit. That said, you can't eat as much as an elephant or a horse. What's the answer? Juicing! The juicer is a great piece of technology that can now pump these micronutrients into your blood without having to wake up your digestive system. I gained a lot of attention early in my journey by walking around with my sunlight juice in a mason jar. Green juice is always a conversation starter.

Non green vegetables like carrots, onions, beets, and turnips can all be used in your salad. They all contain great nutritional value, but they just can't compete with the superhero, and its trusty sidekick.

JUICE VS. SMOOTHIE

Juice is made through a machine that extracts the fiber, leaving you with liquid micronutrients ready to drink and inject directly into your bloodstream. There are centrifugal juicers, and there are cold press juicers. Cold-press juicers are much more expensive because they are more effective, as they squeeze the juice out with force. A centrifugal is more like your teeth, grinding the food up and extracting the fiber.

Smoothies or shakes are done in a blender. This means there is no extraction, which in turn means you are drinking your fiber. Fruit is best for smoothies because it's an opportunity to ingest a large amount of your "superhero." They're great for babies, people who work out hard, and people who are always on the go. They are filling and can be considered a meal replacement, whereas juice is a beverage. The best time to have your smoothie is for breakfast, so that you're "breaking the fast" with not only fruit, but emulsified fruit. Your digestive system will love you for this! I recommend using berries, because it's a very important food, but not too many people eat enough of them because they're small.

Drinking your sunlight is a fantastic way to improve or maintain your health. The question I get asked often is, what's better? Well, one is a car, and one is a motorcycle. They are both different types of vehicles, but either will get you to where you want to go.

SOCIAL MEDIA ASSIGNMENT:

Post pictures of your smoothie. Spread awareness to your audience and inspire someone today.

TAGS: #SunlightSmoothie #ThreeDLife #EatTheSunlight

MAKING A
SUNLIGHT SMOOTHIE

1. PUT 10 OUNCES OF BERRIES IN THE BLENDER
2. POUR NATURAL COCONUT WATER OVER IT UNTIL IT
   ALMOST COVERS THE BERRIES
3. ADD A BANANA
4. ADD A HANDFUL OF A LEAFY GREEN

SUNLIGHT SUGGESTION 1:
SWITCH UP YOUR BERRY TYPES SO YOU GET
THE BEST OF ALL

SUNLIGHT SUGGESTION 2:
USE FROZEN BERRIES SO
YOU CAN STOCK UP

SUNLIGHT SUGGESTION 3:
DRINK YOUR SUNLIGHT SMOOTHIE WITH A STRAW TO
GET THROUGH THE THICKNESS OF IT.

SUNLIGHT SUGGESTION 4:
MAKE THEM WITH YOUR KIDS!
THEY LOVE TO BE INVOLVED

SUNLIGHT SUGGESTION 5:
YOUR SMOOTHIE IS THE PERFECT BREAKFAST
BECAUSE YOU'RE... BREAKING FAST AND WAKING
UP YOUR DIGESTIVE SYSTEM

www.EATTHESUNLIGHT.com

PROTEIN

"Where do you get your protein?" is the most consistently asked question in health. In most cases, the person asking it has no clue what protein is, what it's made of, and how the body works. But they are still quick to speak so passionately about protein. The blind truth is that the need for protein is simply ingrained in their heads. This is classic, state of the art programing.

Protein is a nitrogen-based structure that is composed of different combinations of amino acids. Basic elements of all animal and plant tissue are composed of protein. This makes protein essential to the human body as they repair cells, form enzymes and hormones, produce neurotransmitters for the brain, and are the building blocks for muscle.

The problem is we were trained to think we need to eat protein, and that's just not true. If it were true then how could horses, elephants, and gorillas be so strong? We need to consume amino acids. These amino acids create protein inside of our bodies. And that is the key fact that one needs to know in order to continue the debate: Protein is made inside of us!

Therefore, when you eat second-hand protein, such as flesh, dairy, and eggs, the body has to break it down into amino acids and then rebuild into protein, which wastes unnecessary energy. If that's not enough reason for you, your protein sources must be altered or denatured for you to consume, which makes it foreign to the body. You're the only animal who cooks flesh, soaks and boils beans, and uses pasteurized milk…right?

Look at a cow as an example. It eats greens (first-hand) to be big and strong, and then you eat the cow (second-hand) to be big and strong. The truth is, you will get quality living amino acids from your fruits and vegetables and be able have muscles just fine. Especially with sprouts!

In my book, *Protein Kills: Seven Reasons Why a High-Protein Diet Can Be Deadly,* I go inside the human body and detail all seven reasons. They are:

1. Protein Burns – It's on the acid side of chemistry which causes inflammation.

2. Protein Steals Energy – It's a structure, so the body must do work to break it down to amino acids.

3. Protein Causes Congestion – The body produces more mucus to neutralize the acids.

4. Protein's a Stimulant – Flesh and dairy protein have hormones produced by the animals which in turn stimulate your adrenal glands.

5. Protein Weakens Kidneys – The body does not store protein, so it must be removed through the kidneys, and human kidneys don't handle acids well.

6. Protein Increases Injuries – Putting yourself in an acid state weakens your bones, muscles, tendons, etc.

7. Protein Attracts Parasites – Left over flesh brings forth worms and mixing protein with other foods causes rotting.

WHAT OTHER EXPERTS SAY ABOUT PROTEIN

T. Colin Campbell, PhD

"According to the recommended daily allowance (RDA) for protein consumption, we humans should be getting about 10% of our energy from proteins. This is considerably more than the actual amount required. But because requirements may vary from individual to individual, 10% dietary protein is recommended to insure adequate intake for virtually all people."

Dean Ornish, MD

"Too much protein, especially animal protein, puts a strain on your liver and kidneys and promotes osteoporosis. Too much animal protein, especially red meat, has been linked with significantly increased risks of heart disease, prostate cancer, breast cancer, and colon cancer."

Robert Morse, ND, D.Sc., I.D., M.H.

"Research studies done by some of the world's top universities have proven, over and over again, that meat protein is toxic to us when it is absorbed through our intestinal walls. This creates acidosis; affects an immune response; and invites parasites. In my opinion, high protein diets kill thousands of people directly each year, and thousands indirectly. High protein consumption does not fit our species, nor is it physiologically sound."

Kris Walker, MD

"With aging comes a loss of lean tissue mass, both bone and muscle, approximately 2 kilograms per decade after age 50. Protein is an essential element of muscle and bone, and severe protein deficiency causes muscle-wasting. Studies show a positive association between protein intake and lean body mass. Diets high in protein, however, cause a net acid load in the body and an increased secretion of nitrogen, which can be an indication of muscle wasting; that is, high protein diets are acidogenic, and chronic metabolic acidosis stimulates muscle breakdown. Increased acidosis, with a stable protein intake, causes an increased renal acid load. Protein intake does increase the ability of the kidneys to exercise ammonium to regular acid base balance, but the increased acidosis increases muscle and bone breakdown, and may lead to a loss of lean body mass. A higher protein diet leads to increased urinary nitrogen, partly from muscle breakdown, and partly from the increased ability of the kidney to buffer acid as NH4. As we age, kidney function declines. Glomerular filtration is reduced by 50 percent from age 20 to age 80, and most of this decline occurs after age 50. Day to day, stability of acid base status is dependent on the kidneys' ability to excrete acid."

Gabriel Cousens, M.D

"The biggest fear generated by pro-meat eaters and new vegetarians is about not getting enough protein. The real problem is just the opposite: We take in too much protein. According to the Max Planck Institute for Nutritional Research in Germany, there are many vegetable sources of protein that are superior or equal to animal proteins. The Planck Institute found complete vegetarian proteins—those that contain all eight essential amino acids—to be available from almonds, sesame, pumpkin, and sunflower seeds, soybeans, buckwheat, all leafy greens, and most fruits. Fruits supply approximately the same percentage of complete protein as mother's milk."

Norman Walker, DSc

"The human body cannot utilize a complete protein, such as the meat of animals, fish, or birds, as a complete product, but must break it down and disintegrate it into the atoms and molecules composing it. It then recombines such atoms as are necessary to build up the particular amino acids required at the moment, which may be entirely different from those in the meat we eat. During this process of breaking down and disintegration, the digestive system is really working overtime, which results in excessive quantities of uric acid. This uric acid gets into the body as a matter of course and is absorbed to a great extent by the muscles. Sooner or later the saturation point is reached in some of the muscles, and the acid crystallizes, forming tiny uric acid crystals in the shape of microscopic hard, sharp splinters. It is then that the real trouble begins, because the movement of these muscles causes these tiny sharp points to pierce the sheathing of the nerves and the resulting torture is labeled rheumatism, neuritis, or sciatica, etc."

SOCIAL MEDIA ASSIGNMENT:

We need to wake people up about protein! A twelve-year-old kid recently asked me where I get my protein (the brainwashing has begun). Post your views about protein or quote me to spread the word.

TAGS: #ProteinKills #ThreeDLife #EatTheSunlight

PROTEIN POWDERS

Powder companies are the biggest offenders of exploiting protein to increase business. With the wave of fitness sweeping social media, the protein powder manufacturers have cashed in. All you have to do is go to the gym, and you will see people dumping these unnatural powders into their drinks. It's like powders are the new steroids! Everyone is obsessed with getting big and strong, and they were conditioned to think that powders are the answer.

Whether you're using powder from whey, casein, or soy, they're all isolates! Isolates go through a chemical process in order for the manufacturers to isolate just the protein. Protein isolate is not a whole food and doesn't have the alkaline minerals that are needed to neutralize the acidity of protein. As I've stated in my books and seminars again and again, protein is on the acidic side of chemistry. This is a big reason why, if you look closely at people who consume powders, they almost always have skin problems.

Protein powders are a denatured processed product that will cause an immune response to the body. And don't forget, a lot of them stand the chance of having GMO ingredients. And if that's not enough, these isolates have been processed to remove fat, which promotes the loss of their original healthy properties.

Whether you're dealing with a protein powder that has a slew of ingredients with big words (most of them do) or a raw vegan green powder with one or two ingredients, I recommend you stay completely away from protein powders, bars, and drinks of all kind.

Don't succumb to the powder game; it's another way the establishment takes advantage of a society that wants quick results. And don't forget horses, elephants, and gorillas don't need a protein shake to be strong.

SPROUTS

In the life of a plant, sprouting is the moment a seed comes to life! It's a baby vegetable essentially. This includes beans, lentils, and grains. When you sprout these foods, they then become alive and can be eaten raw!

When the seed germinates, a tail will pop out. This process promotes healthy living. Sprouts actually have more nutritional value than the adult plants. Example. Brocco sprouts have more nutritional value than full-grown broccoli.

Why Sprouts?

1. Sprouts can have up to 100 times more enzymes than uncooked fruits and vegetables.

2. The quality of the protein in the beans, nuts, seeds, or grains improves when it is sprouted.

3. The fiber content of the beans, nuts, seeds, or grains increases substantially.

4. Vitamin content increases dramatically.

5. Essential fatty acid content increases during the sprouting process.

6. During sprouting, minerals bind to protein in the seed, grain, nut, or bean, making them more useable in the body.

7. Sprouts are the ultimate locally grown food. You can sprout at home in a mason jar!

8. The energy contained in the seed, grain, nut, or legume is ignited.

9. Sprouts are alkalizing to your body.

10. Sprouts are inexpensive.

If you like to work out hard and want to fuel those muscles, step up your sprout consumption. The living amino acids in sprouts are unlike any on the planet. Put them in your leafy green salad, make a wrap, or juice them. Sprouts are what your "protein powders" are supposed to be!

HERBS

Herbs or botanicals are a must-have. These amazing plants were put here for medicinal reasons and can help us in so many ways. In fact, the medicines and prescription pills that humans now lean on are derived from herbs (such as in Chinese medicine).

Many herbs are green and leafy, which puts them in the category of "greens," the "sidekick" to fruit. Some of these include parsley, dill, basil, cilantro, plantain leaf, and more. But there are many other plants that can be considered medicinal. Many are barks, roots, and seeds.

Each herb has a purpose and when mixed together by a professional, you have powerful medicine that works, as long as it's paired with the correct diet. An herbal protocol is a major part of healing, making it a pillar of detoxification (more on that later).

I recommend that you find an herbalist near you and get to know them. You can learn the herbs yourself and find an herb farmer as well. That's what I do, as I make my own teas. I recommend the consumption of herbal teas daily, as they are a great way to get these medicinally in your body. Please put down the coffee! Coffee, much like dairy, serves the body no purpose.

ORGANIC VS. CONVENTIONAL VS. GMO

This is one of the most controversial topics in health. Some people say there is no difference, and it's just a conspiracy for organic labels to make more money. Others won't touch conventionally grown foods. I'm glad you're reading this to get my take.

If pesticide sprayed foods kill a bug, why would I want to eat it? If it killed that beetle or worm, what makes me think it won't hurt me? So in my opinion, organic is always better. It just sucks they had to make up the label and jack the prices up. Organic is generally a dollar more.

I want to point out, even though eating organic is best, it's not realistic 100 percent of the time. There are going to be foods shipped to your area that are not available organically. I'm OK with consuming conventionally grown produce if you wash them. My favorite way to do this is by filling up the sink, adding some white distilled vinegar and soaking the food for seven to ten minutes. This helps get the dirt off too.

If you're on a budget, only go for organic produce that does NOT have a thick peeling, such as apples, peppers, and berries. But get conventional foods that DO have a covering, such as melons, oranges or avocados.

I also recommend going to your local farmer's market and getting to know the farmers. Some farmers don't spray, but don't have the title of "organic" because it costs a boatload of money to get the label. You have to ask.

When you're in the grocery store, you should pay attention to the PCU numbers.

5-digit code, starting with a 9 = Organic

4-digit code, starting with a 4 = Conventional

5-digit code, starting with an 8 = GMO

GMO stands for genetically modified organism. This unnatural way of growing food started in 1996 and is known to contribute to poor health. They actually alter the seeds in the lab. My feeling is that you should stay away from these foods altogether. This is the fruit and vegetable version of artificial foods, like candy and margarine. They're altered, man-made, and destructive foods for the human body.

ARTIFICIAL FOODS

How can they make gum that tastes like a burger? How can they make cherry-flavored soda? How can they make Doritos that taste like buffalo wings?

Artificial/processed foods are a prime example of humans messing around and screwing things up for greed. I've had the opportunity to meet lab workers who make a living off of making new flavors and ingredients, and I'll tell you, this is a big business.

Artificial foods can be categorized as almost anything in a box or bag. They are acid-forming because someone is playing around with chemistry.

It's important that you start paying attention to your ingredients; forget the calories, fat, or protein. I teach clients "label laws." Here are your label laws:

1. Five or more hits the door. Anything with five ingredients or more is not quality food (unless sprouted).

2. No words with three syllables or more. If you can't pronounce it, it's not for you.

3. No high-fructose corn syrup.

4. Nothing that is enriched, bleached, or unbleached (super processed).

SOCIAL MEDIA ASSIGNMENT:

Post pictures of your labels! Ingredients are what counts. I want to make sure you're checking them.

TAGS: #LabelLaws #ThreeDLife #EatTheSunlight

DAIRY

Dairy has no place in the human diet! You are designed to drink your mother's milk for the first few years of your life and then be weaned. There is no other animal on earth that drinks milk as an adult. It's a white pus-like fluid from a big, lethargic, enslaved animal, that is meant for a calf. On top of that, in most cases, we lack the enzyme called lactase, which is found in the microvilli of our small intestines and used to break down the sugars in milk (lactose).

Cheese is the worst. It is one of the most acidic foods on earth. I used to be addicted to cheese. I would eat it any way possible. Blocks, shredded, slices, cottage, and grated. I remember finally understanding the truth and saying to myself, "How the heck am I going to get off it? I love cheese!" But the truth sets you free, and I did it. And so can you!

They programmed us with fancy promotion of milk mustaches and commercials throwing around buzz words like calcium and protein. Why isn't the "milk does a body good" campaign still around? Because it was a lie.

I can't tell you how many times I have taken a client off of dairy and saw amazing results. Dairy is mucus-forming, acid-forming and is filled with all sorts of antibiotics and hormones that you are injecting into your bloodstream. What's the point? Dairy is the devil.

Reasons to Not Consume Dairy:

1. Contains unwanted ingredients such as pesticides, hormones, and antibiotics.

2. Cattle are slaves and live stressful lives; this adrenaline and energy is transferred into the milk.

3. Cattle milk is for calves, not humans.

4. The high protein content causes a slew of issues, giving you an acidic environment.

5. Cow's milk contains a very powerful growth hormone, insulin-like growth factor-I (IGF- I). This promotes tumor growth.

6. Dairy is mucus-forming, which leads to allergies, breathing issues, congestion, etc.

7. Cows emit significant amounts of methane, a greenhouse gas even more potent than carbon (about twenty times more).

8. Animal welfare. Cattle are artificially inseminated, and the babies are taken away from the mother. Their udders become sore from the machines milking them. They are true slaves. All for money.

FLESH

Notice I use the word "flesh." Hey, I'm just being honest. That's what it is, isn't it? Meat is another word that we just throw around without any meaning. "Chicken" is the worst in our language. I mean, no one even looks at "chicken" as an animal anymore; it's a product to most. Especially kids. How many five-year-olds do you know who are addicted to chicken nuggets? If you explain to a kid what chicken really is and show them a picture of one, and let them make the correlation, they will flip out! That's because their intuition kicks in, and they know that chicken is a breathing, living animal that has parents. I've seen it happen.

So the controversial question in health is…Are we supposed to eat flesh? My answer is simple. Probably not. Why would you have to cook it when no other carnivore does? There isn't much of a debate that we are frugivores and are meant to eat a mostly fruit-based diet. However, when man migrated up north, we started hunting in the winter months to live. Our ancestors also ate flesh for celebratory reasons (which wasn't every day). So can we eat flesh? Yes. Is it meant for our GI tract? No! Can you rob a bank? Yes! Should you rob a bank? No!

It can be debated that fish are to humans what insects are to primates. I personally don't eat flesh for spiritual reasons, but if that wasn't the case, the only flesh food I would eat is fish. Specifically cold water fish, which are rich in omega 3's, such as mackerel, salmon, or tuna. But, it's still an animal that suffocated to its death, which means it pumped adrenaline into its flesh. And on top of that, it's still a high-protein food that is acid forming. That said, if the ONLY flesh food one were to consume was cold water fish, I would recommend no more than twice per week.

I have a hard time recommending the other flesh foods such as cow, pig, chicken, turkey, and other seafood like lobster, mussels, and clams. However, I have had clients who don't want to give it up. I say to them as I say to you at this moment, bring your consumption level way down. Combined with the cold water fish, eat flesh only two to three times per week. And be ready to add some extra days to your detoxification practice to do some extra cleaning. These flesh foods are highly acidic and damaging to our bodies.

General Food pH Chart

10.0 Alkalinity	Spinach	Carrots
	Cucumbers	Alfalfa Sprouts
	Onions	Celery
	Cabbage	Lemons & Limes

9.0 Alkalinity	Mangoes	Kiwi
	Eggplant	Blueberries
	Figs & Dates	Melons
	Grapes	Pears

8.0 Alkalinity	Apples	Bell Peppers
	Avocados	Bananas
	Almonds	Mushrooms
	Pineapple	Oranges

_7.4_   **_Neutral for the Human Body_**

6.0 Acidic	Milk	Eggs
	Rye Bread	Fish
	Most Grains	Cocoa
	Yogurt	Oats

5.0 Acidic	Chicken	Turkey
	Beer	White Rice
	Most Beans	Cooked Corn
	Wheat Bran	Butter

4.0 Acidic	Coffee	Cream Cheese
	White Bread	Popcorn
	Wheat	Most Nuts
	Beef	Tomato Sauce

3.0 Acidic	Pork	Shellfish
	Cheese	Pasta
	Vinegar	Chocolate
	Soda	Most Artificial Ingredients

HEALTHY FAT

Much like "carbs," sugar, and calories, not all fat is created equal. Healthy fats and omega 3's are key for a well-functioning brain and nervous system. Trans fats and saturated fats can be deadly as they raise your cholesterol and increase your risk for heart disease. Some healthy fat foods are:

Avocados

Olives

Nuts & Seeds

Cold Water Fish

When eating the sunlight, the best place to add in your healthy fats is your salad! You can top your salad with avocado, olives, nuts, or seeds. I am a big advocate of seeds. They add crunch to your salad and are loaded with vitamins, iron, and fiber.

Some seeds I recommend are:

Flax Seeds

Hemp Seeds

Sunflower Seeds

Pumpkin Seeds

Sesame Seeds

Fennel Seeds

Chia Seeds

You can get ground flax seeds and use them as "breading" on some of your dishes. You can use chia seeds to make pudding. You can even grind up soaked sunflower seeds and make a sauce.

While seeds are my choice to top a big sunlight salad, nuts are great for a light snack. Of course, they are better uncooked, and you can always add some sea salt yourself. Another use of nuts can be soaking them overnight (making them softer and easier to digest) and then putting them through a food processor to create a pâté, sauce, or a sunlight dessert. Different variations of grinding soaked nuts can take your recipe game to another level. I recommend using our website for recipes. But just make sure this is moderate, as you don't want to clog yourself up with too much fat!

SOCIAL MEDIA ASSIGNMENT:

Post your sunlight salad and spread this awareness to your audience and inspire someone today. Get heavy with the sprouts and healthy fats. Make it a big one!

TAGS: #SunlightSalad #ThreeDLife #EatTheSunlight

MAKING A SUNLIGHT SALAD

1. LEAFY GREEN BASE - Spinach, Kale, Romaine, Arugula, etc

2. COLORS - Peppers, Cucumbers, Tomatoes, Onions, etc

7. DRESSING - Olive Oil, Lemon/Lime Juice, or Home Made

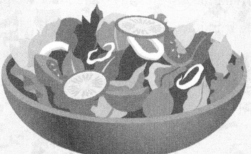

3. KIDNEY FOODS - Dandelion Greens, Beets, Parsley

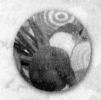

www.EATTHESUNLIGHT.com

6. DRIED FRUIT - Raisins, Dates, Cranberries, etc

4. SUPER SUNLIGHT - Herbs and/or Sprouts

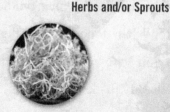

5. HEALTHY FAT - Nuts, Seeds, Avocado

① SUNLIGHT SUGGESTION 1: Cut on time and effort. Find a big Tupperware bowl, fill it up with your Sunlight Salad once per week. Draw from your big bowl to have your daily Salads.

② SUNLIGHT SUGGESTION 2: Use different Herbs and Spices to change the flavor of your Salad. IE - Mexican, Italian, Indian etc.

③ SUNLIGHT SUGGESTION 3: Master the art of making Dressings so you're never bored.

OILS

While oils are technically termed a "healthy fat," overusing oils can be very damaging to the human body. The processing method for industrial oils involves factories, many machines, and chemicals like hexane. It's essentially processed fat and because it's denatured, it creates an immune response in the body. If you cook the oil, it's even worse, as it now becomes a toxic carcinogen. Oils are meant for machines, not our bodies. If you want the amazing perks of olives or avocados, eat olives and avocados, not their oils!

While oils are key for marinades, dressings, and sauce recipes, you can easily replace them by using fruit juice or vegetable broth. Having lemon, apple, or grape juice on hand can help, and you can always make your own vegetable broth. In fact, the broth idea may add more flavor, as you can hand select your own vegetables, herbs, and spices.

To make a vegetable broth, simply throw ingredients like celery, onions, carrots, rosemary, basil, and parsley in a pot. Add just enough water to cover your sunlight and now simmer on the stove for an hour or two until it's the taste you desire. When done, you can then throw your broth in a Tupperware container. Now you have your new "oil" to use for recipes or healthy cooking. You can also buy already made veggie broth.

FOOD COMBINATIONS

The most underutilized and "slept on science" in health is proper food combinations. I see so-called "health gurus" posting pictures of totally wrong combos, and it's very revealing to see who knows what they're talking about and who doesn't.

The pancreas is responsible for putting out enzymes that break down our food. However, not all enzymes are created equal. In other words, the enzymes needed to break down an apple is different than the enzymes needed to break down flesh. When we combine foods, it confuses the body, which will manifest into an unhealthy gut.

We are the only animals on earth that combine food. There is no lion eating a gazelle, with rice on the side. Humans screwed this up. I call it the "Thanksgiving Syndrome." This is where we pile loads of different foods on our plate and spend the next two hours confusing our body, as it tries to break down our abominations.

There are two terms you need to have an understanding of:

1. Fermentation

2. Putrefaction

Both of these terms mean decaying or rotting. Fermentation has to do with the decaying of sugar, and putrefaction has to do with the decaying of protein. Both processes will lead to parasites, bad bacteria, and candida.

SOCIAL MEDIA ASSIGNMENT:

Get two empty plastic water gallon containers. Place a piece of flesh in one and a piece of fruit in the other. Bring both containers to the hottest part of your house (perhaps the attic?). This will simulate the warmth inside your gut. Leave them there, and then go look after two months. Take a picture and upload to social media. I want to see!

TAGS: #Fermentation #Putrefaction #ThreeDLife

The 3 Food Combination Rules:

1. Always eat your fruit alone (unless dried like raisins).

2. Don't mix protein with starches.

3. Greens can go with both protein or starches.

I don't know who came up with the fruit salad, but it's pretty ignorant. If a gorilla comes across a banana tree, it's eating a ton of bananas—it's not mixing with blueberries. Never mix your fruit (unless emulsified aka predigested. IE – a smoothie), especially melons. Melons are so light and soft, they slip right into your intestines from the stomach. But if you block the passage-way with another food, you're going to ferment that melon in your stomach. All you have to do is scan Facebook or Instagram, and you will see "health gurus" posting pictures of fruit salads with melons mixed with other foods.

What else happens during fermentation? Yep, it creates alcohol. I remember my teacher, Robert Morse, ND, telling us a story in class about a guy who ate oatmeal and watermelon as he was rushing to get to his destination. He got pulled over for speeding and was arrested for a DUI because his alcohol level was too high. That's because the body went for the melons, leaving the oatmeal behind to turn into alcohol. Beer is fermented grains, right?

As for putrefaction, starches are long chains of carbon, such as potatoes, breads, or grains. Protein and carbs require their own specific digestive ferment, or enzymes. Being that your body wants sugar (carbon), it's going to digest that first. That leaves the flesh left behind to rot or putrefy. It's very similar to road kill.

Note: Knowing this information, isn't it eye opening that America is obsessed with sandwiches, burgers, and pizza? All three "foods" are starches mixed with protein. Food for thought.

So because of the dead road kill rotting inside of you or the fermenting sugar, you now contain a combination of roundworms, tapeworms, pinworms, whipworms, hookworms, etc. These living organisms that are living inside of you tend to make you hungrier because they are eating your food too. They tend to feed off of your red blood cells, causing anemia. Some tend to lay eggs, which can cause itching and irritability. They tend to give you chronic diarrhea due to your body attempting to cleanse itself. And they also tend to weaken your immune system so you get sick more often.

When we detox someone, the first thing we do is deworm them. Get inside that gut with certain fruits and herbs to get those unwanted organisms out. Once that is done, then we can start correcting the acidic environment. You see, without the presence of material to embed themselves in, many intestinal parasites will not be able to thrive.

So are you going to pay attention to your food combinations now?

WATER

Everyone knows that water is necessary. In fact, the order of survival is…

1. Shelter

2. Water

3. Fire

4. Food

The average person cannot live past three to five days without water. I do NOT recommend trying. Next to oxygen, it's the most important chemistry we need. We need water for many reasons. Here are a few:

1. Helps the body function

2. Removes waste

3. Maintains physical endurance

4. Transports nutrients to cells

5. Keeps body at an ideal temperature

6. Helps move lymph

And more…

I also recommend chugging your water. Have you ever seen a dog drink its water? It doesn't exactly sip, does it? Same with wild animals. They drink when they're thirsty, and when they are, they chug! Unless you're performing athletics or you're working outside, sipping makes no sense.

I advise clients to chug four sixteen-ounce bottles of spring water per day. That comes out to eight cups. If you are heavier than 200 pounds, then you should increase that. Keep in mind though, if you're properly "eating the sunlight", there is quality water in those foods.

Why spring water? Because it's normal. If you were in the wild, is that not what you would drink? Spring water has nutrients in it. If you drink purified water, that only means that the company you're buying from ran tap water through some fancy filter. Distilled water is heated so that the nutrients are killed. The only use for distilled water is for enemas, colonics, and sleep apnea machines. And do I really need to talk about tap water? Isn't it already bad enough we have to use it to clean ourselves? So when you're buying water, make sure it's spring water, and make sure the expiration date is far away!

Another recommendation for clients is to chug their first sixteen-ounce spring water first thing in the morning. When you sleep, you are fasting. Breakfast comes from the term "break fast." The first thing you want to put in your body when breaking a dry fast is water! This is going to benefit you in many ways:

1. Purifies the colon, making it easier to absorb nutrients throughout the day

2. Increases the production of blood and muscle cells

3. Boosts your metabolism by almost 25 percent

4. Purges toxins from the blood, which helps skin stay clear

5. Balances your lymphatic system

So start your day by chugging away! Oh, in case you're wondering, yes it will bring forth a bowel movement. And if it lasts more than sixty seconds, you have more work to do.

DRINKING WITH FOOD

As I've taught you earlier, enzymes break down food and are not created equal. Well, here is something that most don't know. When you drink liquid, it dilutes your enzymes, which hinders digestion. I always teach clients to not drink with their meals; thirty minutes before or thirty minutes after is ideal.

Some of you will have trouble with this, as you have been programmed to drink when you're eating. Your mind thinks you're thirsty, but you're usually not. Especially when you're eating sunlight!

#ThreeDLife
Success Stories

"Personally, the brain fog and lack of focus has been lifted. I definitely have more energy. I've lost thirty pounds, my stomach is flatter, and my waist size has shrunk. This program brought awareness on what I put into my body. Like if I have a stomachache, before it would just be like, "Oh I have a tummy ache," but now I actually can analyze what I did to cause that tummy ache. I don't see myself ever eating meat or dairy again. I was a "cheese-aholic," I loved cheese, but I don't need it anymore. I feel like things are working better inside me. I have a passion toward health now and have even been helping my friends with their health."

-Amy Abo

CHEWING

The most important fact to know about digestion is that it starts with chewing. I used to be a beast! I would chomp my food down like it was race. Oh, the poor pizzas I have devoured in my day!

Slow down! Your digestive system has to do more work if you give it big chunks of food. As you start to chew your food, digestive enzymes found in saliva begin to break it down, preparing for nutrient absorption. You want to receive maximum absorption of all your vitamins and minerals. Enjoy the food, have gratitude; savor the whole spectrum of tastes and aromas that make up the meal.

You can change your chewing habits today. Here are some tips:

1. Count the chews in each bite, aiming for thirty to fifty times.

2. Put your utensils down between bites to help you better concentrate on chewing.

3. Chewing breaks down food and makes it easier on the stomach and small intestine.

4. If under pressure at meals, take deep breaths, chew, and let the simple act of chewing relax you.

5. Don't read or watch TV; keep your concentration on your food.

COOKED VS. UNCOOKED

We have been conditioned to be attracted to cooked food. The smell, the warmth, the satiation. Have you ever noticed that we especially crave a cooked meal in the evening? That's an example of conditioning, as we were programmed to have our big meal when our day's work was over. You know the scenario. The stereotypical man comes home from work and asks his wife, "What's for dinner, honey?" Notice, the right answer will actually excite him.

Unfortunately, when you cook your food, you kill it. In fact, fire changes the chemistry of anything it touches. Just ask a fireman. Fire changes the chemistry of wood, plastic, skin, paper, coals, iron, glass, and most certainly your food. Something as wholesome as onions or peppers are stripped of their nutrients as they burn in your pan or pot. Cooking doesn't add anything, it only takes away. Even boiling foods will deplete the nutrients as the nutrients seep into the water.

Fire changing the chemistry of everything it touches is also an example of why smoking is bad. Everyone knows when you smoke, it produces carcinogens. Guess what? It does with your food too. And if you fry it? Even worse! Potatoes have some good value, until you turn it into your classic French fries or tater tots. Here are some damaging effects of cooking.

HCA's - When you cook flesh, you produce chemicals that contain creatine, which reacts with sugars and free amino acids to form toxins that are linked to numerous health issues, including cancer.

PAH's - Chemicals formed by incomplete burning of carbon containing substances, in foods or fats heated about 392 degrees, including charcoal or browning of foods or any foods fried in oil. These are known mutagens that damage DNA and are linked to diabetes, cancers, and more.

AGE's - Irreversible final products of the Milliard reaction, which is a form of non-enzymatic browning when sugars combine with amino acids. Mainly found when grilling or frying flesh.

Acrylamide - Formed when high carbohydrate foods are heated during long heating processes. They form when the amino acid asparagine reacts to sugars and occurs during baking, roasting, or frying. Potato products are high in asparagine. It is identified as cancerous.

RAW LIVING FOOD

Since the beginning of time, we have been eating raw living foods. As I said earlier, especially fruit, as they come in so many different varieties and flavors. Raw foods are full of living energy, enzymes, and amino acids. Not to mention almost all raw foods are on the alkaline side of chemistry. The more uncooked food you eat, the better you feel and the more your body heals.

As you may have heard in the #EatTheSunlight theme song, our diet is simple. Fruits, vegetables, nuts, seeds, herbs, and sprouts. Why these foods? Because they don't need to be cooked. I'm aware that you may cook them, but as long as it's moderate, I'm OK with it. The point is, they don't have to be cooked, which makes it natural for the human body. Don't you want to eat naturally?

What other foods can be eaten naturally? It's not flesh, for only carnivores can eat raw flesh. It's not dairy because it's pasteurized and cultured so that you don't catch anything. As for eggs, well you can slurp down an egg yolk like Rocky Balboa, but most people would prefer to scramble it or make an omelet. Beans, they're like little stones and need to be soaked for a long time just to be able to be cooked. Grains are not edible until soaked and cooked as well. Have you ever tried eating raw pasta? And powders—have you ever looked at the ingredient list?

Note. When you sprout beans or grains, they then become alive and can be eaten raw! You can find sprouted breads and snacks at your natural health market.

Any food that needs to be cooked is not meant for you. These foods are denatured and hence cause an immune response in your body. This immune response causes a lymphatic reaction, as protective mucus is built up within the tissues and cavities. This protective mucus is needed to buffer the acids, especially in denatured protein. When you start adding this thick mucus, you tend to create the stagnation of your lymph fluid. Again, your lymph fluid is your sanitation department, which brings wastes and acids to the outside world. When the lymph becomes congested, you end up with allergies, poor immunity, and of course, toxemia in certain areas of the body.

THE METHOD

Through my health journey of healing myself and working with clients, I have realized that a 100 percent raw food diet is not realistic to many. I mean, the average American is eating a high-protein diet with heat applied to every meal. That's why I came up with a way to meet yourself in the middle. And that's by simply eating NO MORE than one cooked meal per day. Most people enjoy that meal to be their dinner. So be it.

This method has not only worked with clients, but has worked with random friends, family, and associates who come to me for advice. The one cooked meal per day method can change one's life, especially if you stick to the fruits, vegetables, nuts, seeds, herbs, and sprouts. You can cook and prepare amazing dishes with these sunlight foods. One of the best ways to do so is by marinating them in a Ziploc bag and making a stir-fry type dish. Who said you need chicken, beans, or cheese to have great cooked dishes?

You can marinate vegetables, such as broccoli, kale, onions, mushrooms, carrots, tomatoes, potatoes, and zucchini, just as well as you can a flesh food like chicken or steak. You can create Asian cuisine, Italian cuisine, or Mexican cuisine by just playing around with a Ziploc bag and a variety of herbs, spices, and sauces.

Sometimes I'll just get creative and throw something together. For example, I'll take some beets, chopped parsley, chopped kale, onions, sprouts, water chestnuts, and asparagus and throw them in a bag. Then I will pour in some vegetable broth, lemon juice, horseradish mustard, and oregano. Close the bag and shake it up for a few minutes, then pour into the pan and sauté, adding some sesame seeds to top it off. How easy is that? It takes ten or fifteen minutes, and I just made some delicious sunlight with no oils needed!

If you want to really experiment with flavors, I recommend finding both a local Indian and a local Jamaican restaurant. Try out their "vegetarian" menu and experience how flavorful they make vegetables taste! With ingredients like turmeric, garlic, coconut, coriander, curry, chili peppers, and tamarind, not only are you getting amazing tastes, but you're adding more highly nutritious sunlight to your dish! Instead of rice, pour these flavorful mixtures of vegetables and sauces on a bed of chopped cabbage or chopped beets.

If you're on a budget or you like convenience, stack up on canned and frozen sunlight foods. Now, you still have to follow your "label laws" and be mindful of sodium, but if you shop carefully, you will find quality "non green" canned vegetables like beets, bean sprouts, artichokes, and water chestnuts. For your greens, I recommend frozen kale, spinach, chard, and mustard greens. These are a great for steaming and sautéing. You can even buy your vegetables this way and then use the bulk of your weekly budget to get fresh fruit. Meet yourself in the middle. You can #EatTheSunlight on a budget.

Expand your menu by purchasing a quality food processor. I personally recommend the Cuisinart brand. With this machine, you can slice, dice, and emulsify vegetables, nuts, and seeds. You can really start making gourmet sauces and shredded vegetables that act as grain replacements. These dishes will impress anyone who comes over for dinner.

I promise you, if you learn how to make these recipes, you will knock your family and friends off their rockers when they realize there is only sunlight on their plate. In fact, your family or roommates will come running to the kitchen as the aroma fills up your home. Who knew the sunlight could smell this good, look this good, and taste this good?

The one cooked meal per day method is a must for the diet portion of the #ThreeDLife. If you're consuming more than one cooked meal, you just aren't following along and are depriving your body of the living foods that it wants. In fact, I don't think you should have your one cooked meal if you didn't have your uncooked sunlight during the day. You must earn that cooked meal.

Let's put some regulations on your cooked meal. They are:

1. You're not granted your one cooked meal if you didn't have your uncooked sunlight during the day. It's your medicine and is a must for your body. Don't cheat yourself!

2. Never mix protein with starches (i.e. no beans with potatoes).

3. Aim for leafy greens in your meal four out of seven times.

4. If you don't want to give up your flesh, stick to cold water fish and consume only twice per week.

5. Don't drink with your meal.

6. Follow your label laws.

7. Potatoes and corn are the only starches that are sunlight, but don't consume more than twice per week and never fry them.

8. No dairy. Period.

When guiding clients to an advanced level, I use transitional foods that can contribute to their one cooked meal per day. These foods include:

1. Tofu: If marinated properly, it can really provide great flavor as a flesh replacement.

2. Quinoa: A seed that has a rice texture, it's great as a grain replacement.

3. Hummus or refried beans: Emulsified beans digest better and are great for dipping.

4. Nutritional Yeast: Good for cheese replacements by mixing with oil, lemon juice, and sea salt.

5. Liquid Amino's: Great soy sauce replacement and good for marinating veggies.

6. Olive Oil: Better than vegetable or canola oil, it's good for sauces and marinades.

7. Cold Water Fish: Better than the other flesh foods because of healthy fats.

8. Almond or hemp milk: Better than animal or soymilk, good for sauces.

I want to be clear: The foods I just mentioned are for transitioning or for moderate use only. While they're better than the foods you're replacing them with, they can still contribute to poor health if overused. If you consume tofu once a month, or you use olive oil every now and again, I don't see any problems with that. However, when you feel you're ready to make that next step, I suggest not using these foods. Or you can find some middle ground. Do what works for you.

The rest of your meals are the foundation of your diet, and it's made up of your "superhero" and its sidekick! This is the trick to your health and energy. While people love to make raw food recipes, I believe in keeping your raw foods as natural and simple as possible. In my experience, the smoothie, monkey meal, and salad are the key.

One cooked meal a day…keeps the doctor away!

SOCIAL MEDIA ASSIGNMENT:

Post the one cooked meal that you earned. Spread this awareness to your audience and inspire someone today. I want to see the creativity flow in these pictures. How many ways can you create great healthy sunlight meals? With other people living the #ThreeDLife and looking up the hash tags, you can give or get ideas from each other. Perhaps you can teach me one?

TAGS: #EarnedMy1CookedMealToday #ThreeDLife #EatTheSunlight

SUNLIGHT STIR-FRY
Earn Your One Cooked Meal!

Step 1: Put your sunlight foods in a Ziploc bag

Step 2: Coat the food in vegetable broth or Olive Oil

Step 3: Add your herbs, spices, or sauces

Step 4: Shake bag thoroughly

Step 5: Let marinate anywhere between 5 and 60 minutes

Step 6: Pour into pan and saute' till done

Step 7: You can place your stir-fry over a bed of shredded cabbage, shredded beets, or a steamed leafy green

SUNLIGHT SUGGESTION 1:
Use any combination of sunlight foods, such as, broccoli, carrots, tomatoes, parsnips, beets, onions, peppers, zucchini, kale, mustard greens, water chestnuts, snow peas, green beans, sprouts, nuts, seeds etc

SUNLIGHT SUGGESTION 2:
Use different combinations of herbs, spices, and sauces to create a variety of cuisine flavors such as Chinese, Indian, or Jamaican

SUNLIGHT SUGGESTION 3:
Use your creativity

www.EATTHESUNLIGHT.com

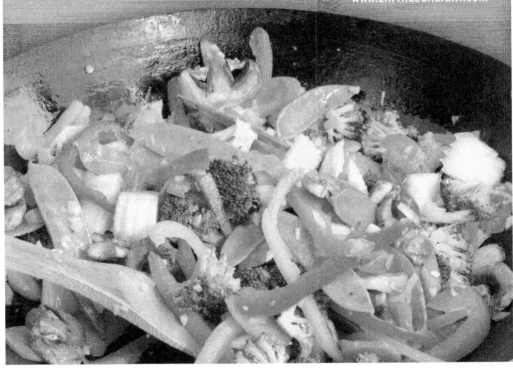

Indian Cuisine Common Ingredients

Potatoes	Red Chili
Cabbage	Turmeric
Coconut	Garlic
Beets	Tamarind
Coriander	Mango
Cloves	Cinnamon
Cumin Seeds (Jeera)	Cauliflower
Fenugreek Seeds (Methi)	Carrots
Fennel Seeds	Eggplant
Green & Black Cardamom	Curry
Mustard Seeds	Onions
Nutmeg	Peas

Chinese Cuisine Common Ingredients

Soy Sauce (Use liquid aminos)

Bean Sprouts

Garlic

Bok Choy

Sesame Seeds

Szechuan Peppercorn

Cilantro

Star Anise

Mushroom

Broccoli

Tofu

Snow Peas

Bamboo Shoots

Hot Mustard

Water Chestnuts

Peppers

Chili

Ginger

Baby Corn

Onions

Jamaican Cuisine Common Ingredients

Plantains	Ackee
Jerk Spice	Calaloo
Yuca	Cloves
Coconut	Allspice (Pimento)
Curry	Bay Leaves
Garlic	Chili
Ginger	Cumin
Guava	Onions
Lima Bean	Rosemary
Pineapple	Saffron
Tamarind	Basil
Thyme	Nutmeg
Yam	Mace

SUNLIGHT SNACKS

Snacks are a part of our society and way of life. Humans love the "snack" and condition our children at young ages to know what a snack is. When you #EatTheSunlight, the key is to not to overthink it. There are plenty of snacks that one can enjoy without it being cooked or escaping the boundary of eating the sunlight.

For the crunchy, salty snack, go with raw nuts and sea salt. Purchase raw cashews, walnuts, or almonds, and sprinkle your own sea salt, pepper, or whatever other spices you want. I recommend counting out twenty to thirty nuts, as you don't want to consume too much fat. Watch your labels; a cooked nut will take away your one cooked meal for the day.

For the crunchy with spice snack, take a crunchy plant food such as celery, carrots, or peppers and dip them in an organic spicy mustard.

For the crunchy with a creamy snack, take the crunchy plant food and dip into an organic hummus. As mentioned earlier, hummus is technically not a sunlight food, so use very sparingly. If you overdo it, you will be giving up your one cooked meal for the day.

Take either a tomato or cucumber and cover it with a variety of spices such as rosemary, basil, and black pepper. If you haven't been overdoing it, perhaps add a bit of olive oil.

Want candy? Get some Medjool dates, and you will feel like you're eating a sweet treat.

HOW MUCH TO EAT?

I suggest eating when you're hungry and not forcing it. This is one of the biggest mistakes Americans make, and it's a classic case of over thinking nature. Your body will tell you when you're hungry and when you're full. Listen to it.

We pick up this "you have to eat" trait from our parents, as parents are so conditioned to force their children to eat. So often a kid isn't feeling good, and the instinct is to not eat (like an animal does in the wild), but the parent forces food down their throat. This is backward. The kid will eat when he or she is hungry again. It's no different than your dog or cat not eating when it doesn't feel good.

Also, how many times one eats per day sometimes depends on how much energy they expended. Perhaps if you do heavy cardio or did lots of yard work, you will eat six times per day. But if you laid around the house all day, you may only eat two or three times per day.

I recommend to always get your monkey meal and smoothie in. I teach clients that this is their "medicine." Even if they get sick of it, still eat it! You must eat your fruit at all costs. This is the secret weapon.

Diet

Daily Menu Example with Six Options:

1. Sunlight Smoothie

2. Monkey Meal

3. Sunlight Salad

4. Sunlight Snack

5. Cooked Meal (if you earned it)

6. Juice or Soup

THE SUNLIGHT STEP-UP

When you master the one cooked meal a day method, you may eventually have the intuition to step up your game to an advanced level. Here are some suggestions:

1. Go from one cooked meal per day to one cooked meal a week

2. Replace your cooked meal with an uncooked meal (raw food recipe)

3. Replace your daytime salad with another monkey meal, and replace your cooked meal with a huge sunlight salad

I am currently working on recipe DVD's and downloads so you can learn how to make great tasting sunlight.

VITAMINS, PROBIOTICS, AND SUPPLEMENTS

I purposely chose not to get into too many details about vitamins (specifically B12), probiotics, and other supplements. I often get asked about these topics when doing live talks and seminars. My answer is always the same. A healthy body does not need anything but simple carbon and oxygen. It's just chemistry.

If you don't have a healthy body at the time, then perhaps you can use vitamins, probiotics, or other supplements as a "bridge" to get to the other side. You should always do what you feel most comfortable with. But I assure you, there is no horse that has a vitamin B12 deficiency because it's a "vegan;" there is no lion that needs to take probiotics for digestion, and there is no ape that needs random supplements. Earthlings just love to over think common sense and make a buck while doing it.

BOWEL MOVEMENTS

This is no one's favorite subject! But I don't give a crap! Sorry, I love corny jokes. When you're eating the sunlight and your GI tract is moving normally, you will begin to poop three to six times per day. Some of you are thinking, "Who the heck has time for that?" But time isn't a problem at all. In fact, your bowel movements will become shorter than your urination movements. You will go into the bathroom, and it will "fall" out of you. You won't need much toilet paper, and the whole ordeal will have taken anywhere from thirty to sixty seconds of your time.

Think about your pet dog for a second. He or she squats and the process takes maybe twenty seconds. And boom, your furry friend is off to the races as it feels light on its feet. We are the dummies that grab a newspaper (or tablet these days) and go hang out in the bathroom for thirty minutes! If you're doing that, then you have serious colon issues coming in your future.

When eating the sunlight for the first time on a regular basis, you may experience nausea or constipation for a month or so as your digestive system adjusts and starts getting ready to clean out! Refer to the detox section of this book. You're going to thank me later.

VEGANISM

I love my "vegan" friends and am super happy that they have altered their diet for the better. And certainly, I'm a big fan of animal rights! However, I think categorizing and labeling people who don't eat animal products hurts the natural health movement.

Now that there's a categorized term for people who don't eat animal products, manufacturers can make money off it. It's only a matter of time before they throw "vegan" stickers on fruit. And if that's not enough, because most "vegans" are so outspoken and proud, it gives off the perception that they're "better" than everyone else. This aggressive righteousness makes it look like a cult, religion, or organization. So now the "vegans" can go to war with the "paleos" and "macrobiotic" folks, who are also aggressively passionate about their "food religion." When will the first grenades go off? In my opinion, we're just going backward.

The biggest problem about being "vegan" is that you can still be unhealthy! Most of the "vegans" never did a proper detox, which means they still have years of lymph stagnation and acids inside of them, creating reason to be unwell in the near future. On top of that, you can still have a poor diet as a vegan!

For example, a vegan could be over consuming starches like pasta, pancakes, and even French fries. Or they could be consuming way too much soy products like tofu, fake "chicken patties" or fake "hot dogs." Or how about artificial snack foods full of oils and chemicals that companies throw a vegan sticker on? How about the protein powder racket for the vegan athletes and bodybuilders? And the same thing goes for the "raw foodists. They could be over consuming raw gourmet desserts or kale chips, which can manifest into poor health too. Usually when this happens, the vegan or raw foodist will then denounce being vegan or a raw foodist because it didn't work. Meanwhile, it's a bad look for the categorizing label that you were so proudly promoting.

This happened with professional wrestler Daniel Bryan. He switched to a vegan diet in 2009 due to an elevated level of liver enzymes and staph infections. The vegans were so proud of him, and he actually got a good deal of publicity off it. But only a few years later, the vegans turned on him because he started eating animal products again. The reason he switched back was because he developed a soy intolerance. With a professional wrestler's intense schedule on the road 300 days a year, I'm sure there isn't many options at the arenas. Then add in the mind conditioning that an athlete needs protein, and I'm sure he overdid the soy foods. This is an example of vegans acting like an over righteous organization, the diet not being specific enough, and someone of notoriety dropping the title because "it didn't work" which is bad publicity. But the truth of it is, Bryan needs to detox and fix his malfunctions of the body and then bring in whatever he wants his lifestyle diet to be.

Through my experiences, I believe that diet needs to be specific and purposeful, and that's where #EatTheSunlight comes in. Mostly fruits, supplemented with vegetables, nuts, seeds, herbs, and sprouts. Let's let these natural foods be in their own category, as they do not need to be denatured to eat. And the beauty is that someone who eats meat, dairy, or grains can still post a picture of fruits or greens and say they're "eating the sunlight." Why? Because they're simply promoting natural food meant for the human body. Isn't that the purpose? To promote health through natural foods? You don't need to be vegan; you just need to #EatTheSunlight.

CLEAN EATING

I don't know who came up with the phrase, "eat clean," but boy is it false. Eating clean would include only eating juicy fruits, because it's the only food that goes through our GI tract effortlessly. But when you look at the pictures of people posting their "eating clean" lifestyle, there's chicken, potatoes, and salmon involved.

Your body doesn't use structures. When your system breaks down structures, it leaves behind "leftovers," which manifests into fungus, parasites, and hardened mucoid matter. Therefore, this "eating clean" trend is a fallacy. I understand what their purpose was—to tell people to cut out the processed and artificial foods. It's just they left the structured, complex foods in there. You don't need to "eat clean;" you need to #EatTheSunlight.

IS DIET BLACK AND WHITE?

Diet and nutrition are funny things. Ten people can tell you a food or diet is good for you, and ten others can make a case that that food or diet is bad for you. However, I think that diet is "black and white," with no gray areas. I don't believe individuality in diet matters, because common sense tells me not to. Your cells, glands, and systems have specific functions; chemistry that enters your bloodstream causes reactions, and what you don't eliminate accumulates. It's that way now, and it was that way two thousand years ago. The only thing that has evolved since then is the technology and society around us.

If you consistently eat acid and mucus-forming foods that cause inflammation and congestion, the human body will malfunction over time, causing problems at the chronic level and eventually degenerative level. If your lymph system is congested and you have an acidic environment inside of you, you are now susceptible to aches, pains, tumors, stones, cysts, rashes, fatigue, weak glands, poor digestion, and immunity. It's just like if all three exits on a strip of highway were shut down, you're going to experience heavy traffic (congestion) and are now susceptible to being late, lots of beeping, people cutting others off, middle fingers being flicked, frustration, road rage, and possible accidents (acidosis). I don't see any gray area; it's all chemistry and certainly simple cause and effect.

All we have to do to realize that diet is "black and white" is look at animals. When they're in their environment and eating the diet they are designed to eat, they are fine. But when we take them out of their environment, enslave them, and consistently feed them foods that aren't meant for them, it manifests into illness. If you consistently feed lions and tigers fruit, they will get sick. If you consistently feed a horse flesh foods, they will get sick.

Carnivores (cats and wolves), herbivores (elephants, horses, cows), omnivores (pigs, chickens, bears, dogs), and frugivores (primates and humans) all have different GI tracts with different levels of digestive acids, which are meant for specific foods. This isn't rocket science. Figure out what kind of GI tract the animal has, and then eat specifically based on that intelligence.

Let's use man's best friend as an example. Dave Ruslander, a veterinary oncologist and past president of the Veterinary Cancer Society said in an article on WebMD:

"Fifty percent of dogs over the age of ten develop cancer at some point. We see malignant lymphoma, which is a tumor of the lymph nodes. We see mast cell tumors, which is a form of skin cancer. There are mammary gland tumors, or breast cancer, and soft tissue sarcomas. We also see a fair amount of bone cancer in dogs."

Sounds like a dog epidemic, yet it's so easily preventable. Dogs are omnivores; they are meant to eat flesh and vegetables, yet we feed them processed "dry" foods, "canned" foods, and milk "bones" with a slew of ingredients. And if that's not enough human error, the average person feeds their dog leftovers from the dinner table, as well as artificial packaged foods like chips and cheese doodles. Why? Because it's cute when they beg? Well, it's not so cute anymore when this member of your family slowly deteriorates in front of you.

Just like the dog's health decreases over time from eating the wrong diet, so does the human's. We see this now more than ever as cancer has tripled since 1980 in human beings. Dogs generally are supposed to live past ten years, and humans generally are supposed to live past one hundred years. But we fall to our addictions and our stresses, as we cut ourselves short of longevity. We just happen to take "man's best friend" down with us.

WHAT IS THE #EATTHESUNLIGHT DIET?

Between the carbon and oxygen needed for our cells, acid-forming foods cause inflammation, and since our GI tracts are almost identical to a chimpanzee's, it was all the common sense that I needed to head down the path to the #EatTheSunlight way of eating.

In order to define this diet, I wanted to group the food instead of grouping the people, to avoid being perceived as a religion or an organization like other labels. I wanted to use the "sunlight" as the key word to promote the foods as "natural" and full of carbon and oxygen.

The foods we are grouping together are alive, do not need to be denatured, and provide our cells with simple carbon, oxygen, and enough amino acids to create superior energy and build healthy protein inside of us. These sunlight foods are:

Fruits
Vegetables
Nuts
Seeds
Herbs
Sprouts

The one cooked meal a day method helps to create a little bit of acid in your diet to balance out the alkalizing living fruits and greens you're consuming. Yet, you're also getting more quality sunlight with herbs and spices. But it's recommended that the one cooked meal a day is to still be the foods grouped above, as you're still eating foods that don't have to be altered, even though you are altering them. It's the concept and principle that matters. You're eating natural foods meant for the human digestive system. You're eating foods in nature that you could pick up and eat. You're eating sunlight.

WHY EAT THE SUNLIGHT?

When you're eating the sunlight (fruits, vegetables, nuts, seeds, herbs, sprouts), you're supplying your trillions of cells with simple alkalizing carbons full of oxygen, which creates vital energy. You will be promoting the movement of your lymph (your sanitation department) so you can bring your toxins and waste to the outside world. You will be strengthening your endocrine glands, which in turn balances your hormones, enzymes, and metabolism. You'll be consuming living amino acids that will form to make firsthand proteins inside of you to strengthen muscle, connective tissue, and bones. And with the proper mindful practices like food combinations, you will be promoting your gut to be free of parasites and fungus. And over time, you will begin to heal, as your body is given the chance to fix and strengthen itself so it can properly digest, absorb, utilize, and eliminate at the efficient level it was designed to operate at.

I understand that there are sick people out there who have gotten better because they have followed someone's "diet." And perhaps that "diet" or "way" is different than what I speak of. So, how did they get better? Well, it's simple. Anytime you increase plant-based foods in the human diet and decrease artificial, processed foods…you get better! Other authors or "gurus" just spin this concept and make it their own because they know you'll improve.

If you take people who eat the S.A.D. (standard American diet), don't feel well, and have chronic issues, and you change up their diet, they will improve. If you put them on the paleo diet, they will feel better. If you put them on a raw food diet, they will feel better. If you put them on the macrobiotic diet, they will feel better. If you slowly take away artificial foods, they will feel better. If you take away dairy foods, they will feel better. It's a given.

However, the individual that got "better" feels "better" because he or she felt "bad" before. If you're in a really bad neighborhood at midnight, this can make the next town look like Disneyworld. If you have a girlfriend or boyfriend who you often fight with, perhaps the next boyfriend or girlfriend will seem like a prince or princess compared to the last. But just because you got better doesn't mean the "diet" you are currently eating is "the one." I don't think it's realistic to have damaged your body for decades with food and then think your new "diet" is "the one" because you feel better on it after a year. Diet is only a part of long-term vitality. So while most people use a GPS (diet) to take you through a series of directions, the #ThreeDLife will just take you straight to your destination (vitality). It will take some time to get there, but at least it's a straight road.

WHAT NOW?

It's time to put this new knowledge to action! I told you what to eat, how to eat, what to drink, when to drink, and all the "why's" you could ever imagine. You were introduced to your "superhero" and its sidekick, the one cooked meal a day method, and should have an understanding of your trillions of cells, and your two rivers of fluids that run through them. But knowing is doing.

You have been programmed to become an addict to many destructive foods, and now is the time to break them. Certainly, the DE-STRESS phase can help with that part.

But I want you to understand, changing your diet isn't supposed to be easy! There will be a learning curve. You may cheat at times. Why? Because you're an addict. Forgive yourself, get back on the wagon, and keep pressing forward. And while you're having that stare down with the bad foods or you're arguing with yourself on whether to order the bad foods, ask yourself, "Is it worth ten minutes of satisfaction?"

I know you'll make the right decision. I believe in you.

INTERVIEW WITH A RAW-FOOD FAMILY

When I was coming up as a health professional and making my name in the Hartford area by doing public speaking, I had the pleasure of meeting Curt Griffing and giving a talk at his venue. Curt owns a company and store called *Raw Food Central (RFC)* where he sells food, hygiene products, classes, and puts on events. Nicknamed the "rawfather," he raised his sons to eat raw. In early 2013, I had the opportunity to interview Curt, along with his son Wynter, twenty-two, who has been raw for eight years and his son Windsor, fourteen, who has been raw all his life. I hope you get out of it what I did.

KWR: Curt how long have you been raw?

Curt: I started a little over thirty years ago when I came down with severe, crippling rheumatoid arthritis, and I had to change my diet and lifestyle to get well, because the doctor said there was no hope for me. He said there was no cure. My knees got as big as balloons; they wanted to replace my joints with artificial ones, and I said, "No way, I want my own joints." So I decided to research health and nutrition, and I came across the raw food diet. I followed it, stuck to it, and I got well slowly over time. Of course, it doesn't go away overnight. It's slow and gradual.

KWR: You raised your children raw…

Curt: Yes.

KWR: Windsor, when you go to school, do the other kids look at you as extreme or weird?

Windsor: I'm homeschooled now, but when I went to school from first to fourth grade, they didn't really care. I was proud of what I did, so they didn't think of me as any different.

KWR: So Curt, did you have to send notes to school?

Curt: I had to talk to the teachers and let them know how we lived. And they were fortunately were very agreeable. They didn't give him things we didn't want him to have. They thought it was kind of neat actually. In fact, they always liked how my kids always ate their food when lunchtime came, and the other kids who had regular cafeteria food barely ever finished their food. It was garbage, you know?

KWR: Oh, I remember. I remember sucking down chocolate milk. So Windsor, you've never had cooked food in your life. What do you feel when you smell it?

Windsor: It doesn't smell good to me.

KWR: Curt, what do you feel when you smell cooked food? You've been raw for over thirty years.

Curt: I mean, what I smell is the seasonings and things like that. If you smell a pizza cooking in the oven, you're smelling the seasonings or toppings, not the dough. I make a raw pizza that's to die for, and people say it tastes just as good, if not better, than conventional pizza. As far as meat goes, that turns me off. Again, you're smelling the seasoning or whatever they put on top of it. But, I've accidently burnt my skin before, and it smells the same as meat cooking on the range. It's a turn-off.

KWR: How old are you Curt?

Curt: I'm fifty-seven.

KWR: So Wynter, you've been raw for eight years. You were raised raw; so what happened from being a raw kid to being a raw young adult?

Wynter: Well, I kind of wanted to be what people considered to be "normal." So, I tried different foods that I've never had before. The taste made me not want to eat the "good" food because I had never tasted anything like that before. Then I started having negative effects. I became overweight, had really bad skin, and it was because of that I wanted to go back to being raw. I was conventional for seven or eight years.

KWR: Curt, did he come to you and say, "Dad, I want to eat regular food?" How did you handle that?

Curt: Yeah, he said he wanted to eat like the others, and he was old enough to make his own decision, so I let him do what he wanted to do. I hoped that he would come back around again because he was gaining weight, and his face was breaking out like crazy. He decided on his own that he wanted to come back.

KWR: Winter, how do you feel when you smell cooked food?

Wynter: It depends. I was never into meat even when I wasn't raw; it just kind of grossed me out. There are some foods that smell really good to me. But I don't remember how they taste, so it triggers no response.

KWR: Yeah, me being raw for thirty years…when I see the fast food commercial, I still remember how it tastes!

Wynter: After eight years, you just kind of lose it.

Curt: There comes a point of no return. There's a point where you smell these smells and think of foods, and there isn't a pull anymore. You think to yourself, why would I want to cook my food when I can have something instantly, like bananas? Why cook? Is the five or ten minutes of chewing and enjoyment worth the harm it's doing to your body?

KWR: How many reversals have you seen in your time, where raw food has completely gotten rid of somebody's suffering?

Curt: Hundreds. It's amazing to hear some of these stories. I've seen arthritis go away, cancers, multiple sclerosis. I saw a girl go from a wheelchair to walking in nine weeks. But there is story after story of high blood pressure, high cholesterol, diabetes, and other common things that I've seen go away with a raw food diet.

KWR: So, do you guys ever go out to eat? There is always social pressure from friends and family.

Wynter: I go out a lot with my friends. But I don't eat. It's just for the social aspect.

Curt: Yeah, going out to eat is more like a social event rather than an eating event. We say go "out to eat," but we're really going out to socialize.

KWR: Right, it's like going to a family event; there is always food. Every time. I don't know who made food the social standard. So, Winter and Windsor, do you guys plan on eating raw for the rest of your life?

Windsor: Yes

Wynter: Yes

KWR: Curt, people can be raw, but be going to these raw food restaurants and sucking down dishes made from nuts and seeds, they clog up their lymph…

Curt: Yeah, we're killing ourselves with too much protein and fats. But naturally in nature, you would eat mostly fruits and vegetables only, and the fats and protein would fall into place. Probably 95 percent fruits and vegetables to a 5 percent protein and fat ratio.

Full Interview Can Be Seen on my YouTube Channel:
www.YouTube.com/KevinWReese

CHAPTER 4

DE-STRESS

WHAT IS STRESS?

Can you hold stress in your hand? Nope. It's not tangible, it's not physical. Stress is a person's response to a stressor, such as an environmental condition or a stimulus. Stress typically describes a negative condition or a positive condition that can have an impact on a person's mental and physical well-being.

I teach clients that stress can be broken into two categories:

1. Fight or flight (acute)

2. External drama (chronic)

FIGHT OR FLIGHT

Fight or flight is pretty self-explanatory. If you were being chased by a lion, your adrenal glands would put out adrenaline, which would give you extended speed and power. Your heart would thump and your blood would pump as you run for your life.

If you were to get into an altercation and you knew you were going to have to get physical, your adrenal glands would do the same. There is something about getting punched that will turn you into the incredible hulk! We've all heard the stories of a mother lifting up a car to save a child who was stuck.

Fight or flight causes a severe reaction to the physical body. While this reaction can assist in saving your life, it does put a major stress on you. That's why the body reserves fight or flight for emergency situations. But if fight or flight happens often, certainly your body will pay for it. Here are some effects of fight or flight stress:

1. Pupils dilate

2. Mouth gets dry

3. Neck and shoulder muscles tense

4. Heart pumps fast

5. Chest pains

6. Palpitations

7. Sweating

8. Hyperventilation

9. Extra oxygen needed for muscles

10. Adrenaline release

11. Cortisol released to depress the immune system

12. Blood pressure rises

13. Liver releases glucose to provide energy

14. Digestion slows or ceases

15. Sphincters close

EXTERNAL DRAMA

While fight or flight is acute (short and intense), external drama is chronic (constant). You've heard the term "life happens"? That's basically it! Drama will come into your life from all sorts of external sources. The top five external dramas are:

1. Financial drama

2. Work drama

3. World drama

4. Responsibility drama

5. Relationship drama

All five of these external dramas can stimulate your mind to either create a fight or flight response or cause anxiety and worry. Both stimulate and work your adrenal glands and slow down your lymph through a process called innervation.

This external drama can manifest over time and result in very poor health. Again, you do NOT want to stimulate your adrenal glands to that capacity, and you do NOT want to stagnate your lymph fluid for reasons I taught you earlier. Here are some other effects from external drama:

1. Tense muscles

2. Hyperventilation

3. Release of cortisol, causing belly fat

4. Binge eating

5. Nausea or vomiting

6. Hindered digestion

7. Diarrhea or constipation

8. Anxiety attacks

9. Hair loss

10. Hindered reproductive system

11. Headaches or migraines

12. Lymph stagnation

13. Depression

14. Mood swings

15. Various musculoskeletal conditions

16. Insomnia

You know the feeling…

Seeing those monthly bills, not knowing how you're going to pay for them. Getting up and going to a job you don't want to go to. Watching the news or your social media timelines and seeing all the horrible crimes, conspiracies, wars, and economic woes play out in front of you. Having the overwhelming feeling of having to take the kids to their activities, make dinner, and work your regular job. And last but not least, having a significant other, family member, or co-worker that you don't get along with and end up holding resentment toward.

Yup. Constant external drama. You're familiar?

Well, I have horrible news…

External drama will never go away! It will always be there, and there is no way to avoid it completely. It's a part of human life!

But I have great news too…

You can learn how to handle the external drama and drastically limit the deadly effect it has on you.

Want to know how?

THE UNTRAINED MIND

Your mind is like a dog. It can be relaxed and timid, or it can be excited and hyper. When someone comes to your house, dogs tend to get excited and hyper. They sniff, they jump, they bark, some may even show their teeth. The owner usually exhausts some energy yelling or reprimanding their dog to "knock it off" or "go lay down." A trained dog will follow the instructions of their master and an untrained dog will not. Your mind is no different. What I'm telling you with this analogy is…YOU ARE NOT YOUR MIND. Everyone has a "dog" inside them and a "master" inside them.

Dogs learn through classical conditioning. Don't you remember Pavlov's dog from class in middle or high school? A bell was rung every time the dog was fed. Soon, the dog associated the bell with its food. And eventually, they could ring the bell and the dog would salivate and come running thinking it was food time, even if they didn't put out any food.

Your mind is classically conditioned to crave pizza, ice cream, coffee, soda, television shows, sex, video games, and more. And because that "bell" has been "rung" for so long, it now triggers a response to your body, which makes you crave what it is that your mind has been conditioned to crave. The great news is that unlike Pavlov's dog, you have a higher intelligence and can break these cravings or desires.

I am writing a book entitled *Freedom Has No Cravings: The Guide to Breaking Any Addiction,* which will dissect this in great detail using my own experiments over the years with myself and clients. However, at this present moment, we are on the subject of stress, and I tell you, external drama is similar to cravings. It is an emotion that comes from your untrained mind.

EMOTIONS

Emotions are a natural instinctive state of the mind, which derive from one's circumstances, mood, or relationships with others. They can often overwhelm us, which triggers a physical reaction. The amazing part about emotions is that there are different steps to each one, and they will manifest and turn into a higher state of the original feeling. Here are some examples of emotional levels....

Level 1 -----> Level 2 ----->Level 3

Annoyance -----> Anger -----> Rage

Serenity -----> Joy -----> Ecstasy

Pensiveness -----> Sadness -----> Grief

Distraction -----> Surprise -----> Amazement

Apprehension -----> Fear -----> Terror

Acceptance -----> Trust -----> Admiration

Interest -----> Anticipation -----> Vigilance

Conflict -----> Disgust -----> Loathing

Level three of emotions is really where the physical body is deeply hurt as the external drama turns to internal trauma. We never want to achieve this level of emotion in the #ThreeDLife.

Let's use traffic as an example since everyone can relate to it. You leave your house on time, you're all prepared for your day, and as soon as you hit the highway, you notice there is a traffic jam. You're stuck! You feel annoyance. After fifteen minutes when you realize traffic is not moving, you begin to get angry. Now you have to call your job or the person you're meeting and tell them you're going to be late. Now forty-five minutes have passed and you've barely moved! At this moment, any little thing, such as someone beeping at you or cutting you off, can set your untrained mind into a rage! Hence the term "road rage."

Speaking of the driving, I had a client who was having anxiety attacks every time she got on the highway. The root cause was fear. Fear is a very destructive emotion. In her untrained mind, she developed an apprehension that made her thoughts race. The more it raced, the more fear built up, and when she got on that highway, the terror would flow, bringing forth an anxiety attack. Now she has to pull over to catch her composure. The next emotion she felt not only at that moment, but in her daily life, was sadness. This was due to suffering from this chronic issue and feeling hopeless. And of course, sadness can turn to grief. So with this case, you're dealing with two major emotions. Both having a tremendous negative effect on her physical body.

Here's another one. For lunch at your job, a brand new pizza joint sends over a bunch of pies for the office. You only have two slices; after all, you don't want to look like a pig. As it turns out, this is some of the best pizza you have ever had! You experience serenity. Your mind stays with that emotion and keeps thinking of having more of this pizza as the day goes on. Your workday ends, you get in the car, and while you're driving you say, "screw it" and decide to stop and get a pizza for yourself. As you drive home, the aroma of the pizza fills the car and you begin to get excited. Serenity has now manifested into joy. You can't wait to get home to turn on ESPN and tear this awesome pizza up! Finally, it's here. The TV is on, you have your drink, your napkins, and slice number one goes in your mouth. And at that moment, your joy just turned into ecstasy.

Things that bring forth ecstasy are not good for the body either, as this is how your untrained mind becomes addicted. Just ask a drug addict. Every time they get their drug of choice, they feel ecstasy, over and over and over again. You can break ANY addiction with the training of your mind. I know because I have done it, and continue to word towards ultimate freedom.

THE TWO PARTS OF YOUR MIND

What does a car do? It drives. What does a CD do? It plays. What does a camera do? It records. What does your mind do? It thinks!

Thinking is a human being's gift and curse. In order to understand thoughts, it's important to wrap your head around the two parts of the human mind and their functions. They are...

1. Memory

2. Ego

MEMORY

Memory can be compared to a hard drive. Something happens in your life, and that feeling and occurrence gets stored in your mind. You could've been attacked by a swarm of bees when you were ten-years-old, and now every time you see a bee, you're scared. You could eat nachos and cheese every time your favorite TV show is on, and now even when "dieting," nachos are in your thoughts when this show comes on. You could have had a sexual experience, where a certain song was on, and now you think about it every time you hear the song. You could have a deceased parent who was into gardening as their hobby; now every time you see gardening on TV or while out and about, you think of your deceased parent. This hard drive is amazing, isn't it?

Your memory is directly attached to your five senses. These are:

1. Sight

2. Hearing

3. Touch

4. Smell

5. Taste

So now, when you experience one or more of the five senses, it can trigger a memory, which then creates an emotion. You can have a memory that creates one of the five senses. Like the pizza example earlier, the thought of tasting that great pizza brings on sight, smell, and taste memories. Even without having the physical pizza, those memories are there. I haven't had steak in five years, but I can still taste it. When a Taco Bell commercial comes on TV, I can still taste it too. These are forever in my memory as they are yours.

EGO

The problem is, we use the term "ego" as slang. People throw the word around as if it's a replacement for terms like "confidence" or "arrogance." But ego is much more complex than the way people use it in their normal language.

You see, your ego is based on image. It attaches to certain desires, which may include success, validation, and approval. The human ego is often the cause of many hurtful emotions in one's life. Let's explore.

If someone were to tell you that you're ugly, your ego would be bruised, and it would create an emotion. Either sadness, anger, or both. It could even manifest into you becoming self conscious, which in turn could create all sorts of lifetime complexes.

If your father never complimented you or gave you praise, your ego will seek it. You will try your hardest to show off to get what you're looking for and maybe even act out when you don't get it. And by constantly seeking it, you will set yourself up for failure every time as the cycle of sadness, disappointment, and anger manifests into resentment.

"The ego is not who you really are. The ego is your self-image; it is your social mask; it is the role you are playing. Your social mask thrives on approval. It wants control, and it is sustained by power, because it lives in fear." - Deepak Chopra

Have you ever been broken up with or been turned down by someone you like or love? Most of us have. We often refer to it as "heartbroken." This is a major bruise to the ego, which causes a slew of emotions that can manifest into grief.

This can turn to depression as you wonder why this occurrence happened and what you did wrong. Sometimes it takes years to heal from this. The ego won't let it go.

Have you ever been obsessed with a material item? That new BMW? The big house in the nice neighborhood? The super sexy girl who looks amazing in that bikini? This is ego as well, as it craves nice things to validate your success.

Ego can also be your friend though, for the ego is completive! Michael Jordan, Joe Montana, and Wayne Gretzky all contained a level of competitiveness that drove them to be the best in their sport. That's ego. There's nothing wrong with that, as long as one can turn it off when they go home. That's the key. The untrained mind will think and think and think, and the thoughts will eat at you. Getting knocked out of the playoffs or missing a shot can be devastating to the ego. Of course, this external drama will result in poor health, just as the other examples will.

You probably thrive to be the best at your job too. Whether you're an electrician, a dentist, or a teacher, I'm sure you want to be better than your associates and you desire to make more money. But at the end of the day, does it truly matter? The sun will still come up and the wind will still blow no matter how much money you make or how good you are. So I say, thrive to be the best, but train your mind to turn it off when you step off the playing field. Your health depends on it.

THE BALANCE

In case you're wondering, this is why monks, Sufis, and mystics wear what they wear and live their strict lifestyles. One of their purposes is to eliminate ego to get closer to the natural source. In doing so, one rids themselves of regular attire, traditional living, and usually their hair. Understandably, it's not for everyone. Most humans enjoy competition and all sorts of material items. Again, the problem comes from not having a trained mind to balance the two worlds.

Mahatma Gandhi is a great example of someone who thrived at training his mind, yet used his ego to his advantage.

Gandhi became the greatest activist perhaps we have ever seen. An attorney with great earning potential, he went in a different direction and started representing those who needed his help. Eventually he dropped his profession all together and focused on his calling. He was outspoken on animal rights, racism, violence, and ultimately his life's work helped free an entire nation. He had the most profound ripple effect we have ever seen outside of spiritual leaders like Buddha and Jesus. He inspired the likes of Martin Luther King Jr., Nelson Mandela and John Lennon, who in turn inspired millions more.

He lived by his own code and essentially wrote the blueprint to training one's mind. He wasn't a monk who lived in the mountains, yet because he lived differently than most, he seemed to be like one. His experiments included owning and traveling with only a few items, eating a strict high-fruit diet, having no sex, making his own clothes, and practicing meditation. But like an athlete bent on winning a championship, he was bent on letting the world know that violence was not the answer. The balance he maintained with his ego is nothing short of remarkable.

A man told Buddha, "I want happiness." Buddha said, "First remove 'I;' that's ego. Then remove 'want;' that's desire. See, now you are left with only happiness."

I know a man whose ego was recently bruised. He was a very proud tradesman. He was looked up to at his job, and his image was that of a respected leader. Well, after thirty years with his company, he had to go on short-term disability for health reasons. His goal was to heal and then come back. However, when his leave was over, they did not take him back. They kindly thanked him for his service and asked him to come clear off his desk. The next month or so, he experienced pain. He didn't understand why, but I did. His ego was attached to his career, and he was not able to walk out on his own terms. His image was taken away.

Very truly I tell you, one must be willing to give it all up. If you have a BMW that you flaunt, you must be ready for it to be taken away. If you are in love, you must be willing to let that person go. If you are great at your career, you must be willing to walk away at any time. This is all attachment. And what we're attached to will cause much pain when we are forced to become unattached. You can still have these things, but train your mind to handle the eventual loss. And I guarantee, there will be loss.

YOUR MIND IS YOUR SERVANT

I mentioned earlier that you are not your mind. What I mean by that is, your mind is a tool, a servant if you will. It's similar to your legs. Your legs are tools that allow you to walk, run, jump, and kick. And your mind is a tool to think, learn, and store data.

When you have to do math, you need to use your mind to add and subtract, right? When you're faced with a challenge, you need your mind to think of a solution, right? As I write this book, my mind is doing work to make my thoughts translate to paper, right? The mind is one heck of a tool, isn't it? But we often let our minds get out of control. Imagine if you didn't have good control of your legs, and they just walked where they wanted.

Have you ever been somewhere and you had a feeling that you were in a dangerous place? Have you ever met someone, and their energy felt off to you? Have you ever done something wrong and then felt bad about it? Have you ever meditated and felt energy rush through your body?

These feelings are from your master. Your master is also known by many as your soul, your spirit, or in some cultures, your heart. The master brings forth intuition, consciousness, purpose, and the feeling of doing right or wrong. Your master is the boss, just as when you get into a taxi in NYC. You tell the cab driver where you want to go, and he drives.

Many times the master and driver will argue. Example: Have you ever had an overwhelming feeling that the way you're eating is wrong and you need to change? But yet, a few hours later you convince yourself that you can have one more candy bar? Your master (passenger) was sending you a message, but your mind took over and convinced your physical body to go get more junk food. This is an example of your mind being your master and not your servant. It's supposed to be your servant, your tool.

Before learning to train your mind, you must understand how the system works. In teaching that, I give clients a very simple tool. The analogy of an old style horse and carriage. It is as follows:

Horses = Emotions
Driver = Mind
Carriage = Physical Body
Passenger = Master

Let's put it all together now.

If you're at work and a co-worker tells you that you're not very good at your job, you're going to feel something, right? Anger, sadness, or both? Now those horses (emotions) can keep going straight and steady, or they can get out of control. In getting out of control, they move, shake, and can send the carriage (physical body) off road even. This affects the carriage (physical body) and can damage it. But you don't have to let the horses (emotions) get out of control. You see, it depends on your driver (mind), as your driver (mind) drives the horses (emotions)!

So I tell you, trace it back to your mind and figure out if it's coming from memory or ego. In the "at work" example, it's ego, right? Knowing where the emotion is coming from makes the world of difference because you're aware now. This awareness can give your master, the passenger sitting in the carriage, a smooth ride.

When I was a kid, I would trick my dad into getting takeout food. It didn't take me long to realize that he was a food addict like I was, so all I had to do was plant a seed. He would come home from work and read the paper, then I would come in and say something like, "Dad, don't you think a pizza would be really good tonight? How about extra crispy in the oven like you like it?" He would look at me and shake his head "no." Thirty minutes later, he would ask me to call the order in. You see, all I had to do was plant that seed, which conjured up a memory, and the memory caused a craving. Perhaps just reading this, you can taste pizza.

The key in training the mind is to let emotions pass. To not let annoyance get to anger, and even if it does turn to anger, to not let it go to rage. If you ever reach level three on any emotion, one needs to put in more training. Once you stop reacting and stop letting yourself get to level two or three, the mind will start becoming trained through classical conditioning and your horses will be in line.

This takes much practice and certainly can't be accomplished in a month. But once you get there, your physical body (carriage) will not go through the trauma explained earlier; your mind (driver) will keep the horses in check, and your master (passenger) will be one happy traveler. In doing this, you will start to hear your master more as your intuition, consciousness, purpose, and the feeling of doing right or wrong will all increase. Has anyone ever told you to listen to your heart? That's what it truly means.

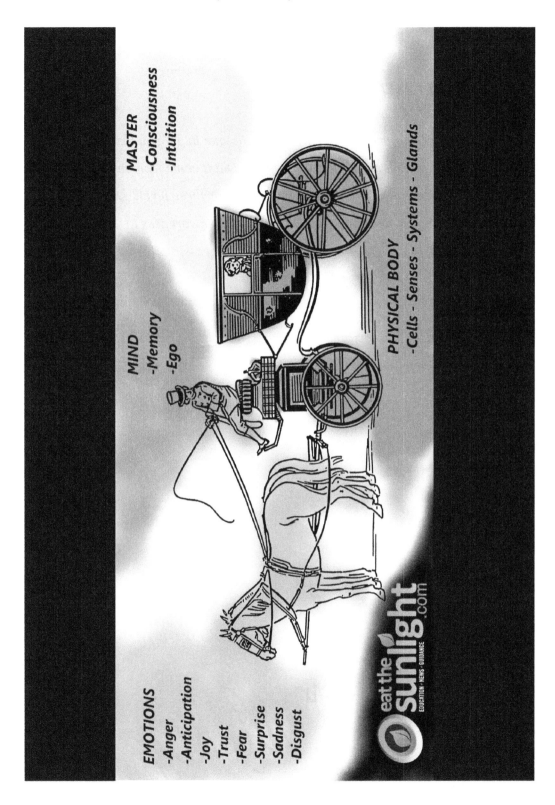

SOCIAL MEDIA ASSIGNMENT:

Post how you used your horse & carriage technique to get you through a situation. Trace the emotion back to the mind. Did it come from memory or ego? Did you stop the emotion to reaching a level two or three level? Did you keep your horses going straight and steady? Spread this awareness to your audience and inspire someone today. I want to see your progress.

TAGS: #TrainingMyMind #DeStress #ThreeDLife #EatTheSunlight

MEDITATION

In training the mind, listening to your master, and relaxing the body, nothing matches the practice of meditation. Meditation is the act of sitting still, silencing your mind, and raising the energy frequencies of the body. It's about pulling the horse and carriage to the side of the road and telling the driver (mind) he has some time off.

It's important that we use the word "practice," as it will take time to work on it. It took me three years to get my meditation practice down, and I still strive to get better at it. The mind is conditioned to do lots of thinking, so telling it to "shut up" can be challenging. But when it happens, it's magic!

Meditation is very much about breathing. During your practice, it may be hard to shut the mind off, or even when you do, a thought or two may pop up. When that happens, you recognize the thought, then bring your attention back to your breath, which in turn silences the mind again.

Concentrate on your inhale and exhale as you drift off into your zone. I teach clients to envision a violet/purple smoke that you inhale and exhale. This gives the mind something to do and violet/purple is the color of third eye chakra. Sometimes when you hit that zone, you will actually see purple, even with your eyes closed.

If you're into prayer or just want to talk to your higher power, before meditation is a great time to do so. By doing this, your intention has been put out to the universe and now your master can receive messages. Listen for the "whispers of the heart," and see where you are guided.

The deeper you get into your meditation practice, the more vibrations you will start to feel. This is because your frequencies are increasing. Remember, we're made up of energy. Everything living is energy. Always remember that. If you're "eating the sunlight" especially lots of fruits, you have a better chance of receiving this amazing feeling, as fruit raises that frequency because of their electromagnetic properties. Many times the bridge of my nose will tingle when meditating. It means one is tapped into the natural energy source that is the universe.

If not for spiritual reasons, meditation is great for the body. Some of its positive health effects are:

1. Decreases levels of cortisol

2. Balances emotions

3. Loosens up your vessels, helping to move lymph

4. Releases tension in the muscles

5. Causes mental clarity

6. Increases fertility

7. Lowers blood pressure

8. Anti-inflammatory

And more…

Anytime is a good time for meditation, but there are two best times for it:

1. When you're emotional

2. Just after waking up

When you're emotional, and your horses seems to be getting a little hasty, meditation can bring you back. Go to another room, or place where you can be alone for five to ten minutes, and meditate. You will be giving your driver (mind) a chance to bring the horses (emotions) back to a slow and steady and pace. This is key in the #ThreeDLife.

For your daily practice, I recommend clients to try it directly after waking up in the morning. This is because your mind is still in a dream state and you are more apt to relax and shut the mind off. Climb out of bed, sit on the floor or on a chair with your back straight and your palms facing up on your knees.

You can start with five minutes and work your way to fifteen or even forty-five. My spiritual teacher wakes up with the sun everyday and spends a few hours with his prayer and meditation practice. He's an example of someone who has been practicing for a long time and is completely dedicated to his practice. I myself go through spurts. Sometimes I can do thirty minutes and others just five. But making the effort and always practicing is what is truly important.

My best meditation usually comes before I do a live speaking appearance. I always drift off into my zone and quiet my mind. Often, I go longer than I would have ever guessed. What felt like five minutes was really thirty minutes. Then, when it's time to grab the microphone, I am completely energized and tapped into the natural source. It's an amazing feeling.

I encourage you to start your meditation practice today. If morning isn't good for you, then find a time that is, and practice everyday around that same time. You will get better and better as you keep going, and you will improve your life greatly. Meditation isn't just a big part of de-stressing—it's the foundation.

#ThreeDLife
Success Stories

"Grateful is a huge understatement for how I feel about the program and how it has changed my life. At the time I started, it was mainly for the detox portion of the program. With all of the horror stories we hear more and more about the foods we eat combined with the toxins being put into the water and the air we breathe, we are constantly put at the risk of developing cancer; to top it all off, I was a smoker. I smoked for twenty-four years and quitting finally seemed like a lost cause in my mind due to having failed so many other times with gum, patches, chantix, etc. Well, thanks to the program, I haven't touched a cigarette in over a month without any substitute chemicals! I thought I simply did not have the willpower to do it, but by utilizing the tools provided in this program, I have become so much more emotionally and mentally balanced. I would have to say that meditation and yoga have been the most useful for me in my day to day life. Like anyone else, I have tons of random issues that come flying toward me at any given time. Had I not been taught how to react accordingly, I definitely would still be extremely unhealthy and headed nowhere fast. And as a mom, that was far from where I needed and wanted to be. Now I'm glad to also be able to pass my healthier habits down to my children. The benefits have been endless, and I could go on all day!"
-Monika Grylls

SLEEP

Sleep is a no brainer, yet many of us just don't get enough of it. We live in an instant society where we have sources of entertainment at the palm of our hands at all times. And this includes late at night. Often, social media or playing on the Internet messes with our sleep.

I've known folks who only get two or three hours a night and think they'll be just fine. This is false. The body needs to regenerate, and sleep is when this process happens. Let's say you have a broken leg. That broken leg is going to do a great deal of healing when you're sleeping.

I had insomnia in my twenties, and I understand how frustrating it can get. I used to have a "go-to-breakfast" that I would eat around 5:00 a.m. on the nights I couldn't sleep. I would be out like a light around 6:00 a.m. because of the sugar crash. It was three scrambled eggs, a can of corned beef hash, two slices of bread with cream cheese, and a glass of orange juice. It would knock me out every time! And yes, the taste is forever in my mind stored as a memory.

I was putting a major strain on my body, not only because of what I was eating, but because the body now has to do a lot of work to break down the food. Hence, eating before sleeping is one of the worst mistakes humans make. In fact, if you eat a light dinner, your body will do more healing while sleeping. Otherwise, it's going to put its energy toward digesting your grub. It goes back to the old saying, "Eat lunch like a king and dinner like a peasant."

Another problem we have with sleep is when we do it. Humans are designed to be up with the sun and sleep with the stars. But a lot of you have third shift jobs and your sleep patterns are all messed up. I understand you're doing what you have to do to make a living, but this is very unhealthy. Again, we are frugivores (primates). Primates sleep at night, and so should you.

One of many factors that played into me quitting my radio job was the time slot. My show was from 9:00 p.m. to 3:00 a.m., and once my lifestyle switched, I was having a hard time with the hours. I didn't want to be going to bed at 4:00 a.m. I desired to go to bed around 11:00 p.m. and be up around 7 a.m. That is ideal.

Not getting enough sleep can manifest into very poor health. Such negative effects are:

1. Impaired attention

2. Impaired alertness

3. Impaired memory

4. Risk for heart issues

5. Risk of high blood pressure

6. Risk of stroke

7. Risk of brain and nervous issues

8. Decreased sex drive

9. Decreased immune system

10. Promotes weight gain

11. Promotes agitation during the day

12. Promotes depression

I often recommend a sleep mask. Your pineal gland is the gland that puts out melatonin when you sleep. But when you wear a mask, you are making your vision completely dark, which causes the pineal to increase more. That said, a sleep mask is much safer and reasonable than taking a melatonin tablet.

Some white noise can certainly help. This day and age, we have our phone and tablets, so all we have to do is find a podcast or app that has some relaxing sounds. Perhaps the sounds of a beach, a rainforest, or the rain will help you fall into your trance. You can also put a timer on these so they turn off after you are asleep.

A breathing exercise that is ideal for nighttime is called the four-seven-eight. You very simply inhale through your nose for the count of four, hold your breath for a count of seven, and then exhale through your mouth for a count of eight. Repeat this four to six times and you will become relaxed. You can also perform this exercise when feeling stressed out.

I recommend you get a full seven to nine hours of sleep. And good sleep! In order to increase the quality of sleep, I have a nightly routine I give to clients. You must dedicate the hour before bed as your new bedtime routine. Here is what you do within that hour:

1. No TV, videos, reading, or Internet during the hour

2. Have a cup of herbal tea (chamomile, lavender, and valerian promote relaxation)

3. You may do some yoga

4. Write a page or two in a journal about how your day went. What did you learn? What could you have done better?

5. Perform your new four-seven-eight breathing exercise

6. Try a sleeping mask and some white noise to help with your quality of sleep

NEGATIVE THINKING

The mind is powerful. What and how you think truly does affect your life. Typically negative thinkers are met with constant "bad luck." You see, your thoughts typically become your words, and your words typically become your behavior. Your behavior typically becomes your habits. Your habits typically become your values. And your values typically become your future. I learned this from Gandhi.

You can point out your negative thinkers when you hear phrases like this:

1. I don't have a choice

2. I can't

3. I missed my chance

4. My goals and dreams can wait

5. They're probably right, so I must be wrong

Or, they just get on social media and complain about everything. Maybe they have no one to talk to, so they vent on social media, or they are seeking sympathy. In fact, I'm going to go to my Facebook timeline right now and pick out some posts that are negative and copy and paste them below. They will be unaltered, so grammar will be messy. This won't take long:

Example 1:

When I'm stressed ever since I was young, I always went running. Today is a super stressful day so I decided to go for a run. Felt a pop in my calf. had to turn around and walk home. Looks like its the elliptical machine instead. #heavyheart

Example 2:

I'm sorry I have to say this.. Ppl want my girl Beyonce to act like black trash and fight in a elevator because her "sister" wants to jump out of character for a sec! for what? Now peep the chicks that are saying this.. how many baby daddies do have? Married? will they ever be? classy? money? Educated? no all across the board NOOOOOOOOO... grow up ppl!

Example 3:

I'm at the dr right now and this guy is not trying to wait so reception is saying he'll get charged and this guys like oh well the state will pay for it. GTFOOOOO ignorant assholes. But receptionist told him ummmm no you'll have to pay for a no show. Entitled ass people.

Example 4:

My ex is such a loser. He wants to see me but still can't man up to apologize. Boy bye! When u become a man maybe I'll think about conversing until then go head...

Example 5:

Thank you to my friends and very few family members that stay in touch, check in, reach out, or just say hi. I really appreciate it and for those that don't respond or reach out anymore, such as... have a nice life. #YouKnowWhoYouAre #FunnyHowThingsChange #ImOnlyHuman

Well, there you have it. Social media is our new soundboard as the negativity flows. These people usually don't sleep well, have anxiety, get sick often, and have rocky relationships. They classify as "poor me's." This is not part of the #ThreeDLife.

SABOTAGE

We're all familiar with sabotage. Some of you have made a life of it! Sometimes when you're doing good, you decide that you want to make it worse. Perhaps you're just not used to doing good, so you jump in and break up your own momentum. And after you stop yourself from thriving, you then wallow in the sorrows that you just created.

Many of you argue with yourself before the sabotage takes place. How do you argue with yourself anyway? Are you two people? I had a client tell me the other day that she had the takeout pizza menu in her hand and she stared at it for a good twenty minutes before pulling the trigger and ordering. After her ten or fifteen minutes of satisfaction (eating), she then felt horrible as she knew what she did was "stupid." And what happens after we cheat? We cheat more! It causes a snowball effect because now your mind (driver) can convince you (the passenger) that you messed up anyway and you might as well keep going. This promotes the horses (emotions) to get all out of control and of course affects your carriage (body).

If sabotaging yourself isn't enough, you can have outside "sabotagers" too! Unfortunately, many times this is done intentionally. Sometimes a significant other will bring home a "goodie" for you when they know darn well that you're trying to change. This is usually done out of control. Perhaps they want to see you unhealthy or fat so they can keep you around. Don't let their insecurities bring you to their level. You're in control, not them.

In many cases, it's a roommate. That roommate could be your significant other or perhaps a parent or child. Someone that you live with who makes food you don't want to eat anymore. You are forced to smell it and see it. Unless you move, you're going to have to deal with it. Use your horse and carriage to guide you through it. Leave the room or the house if you have to until you're ready to be a leader.

Some of you feel obligated to cook for your significant other, even if you're trying to eat differently. A client once told me that she was "old-fashioned" and felt the need to cook for her boyfriend. We were running her through a detox, and she was cooking flesh foods for him! That makes no sense as she was setting herself up for failure. That's like an alcoholic getting behind the bar and making people mixed drinks for others. I recommend having a heart-to-heart talk with your significant other to explain your vision and goals. If they have your back, they will have your back. Period.

It's important to know that you, the passenger (master), is in control, not the mind (driver). Keep up on that awareness and keep practicing it, and good things will start to happen. Soon you will become a leader and the smells from the foods you used to eat will become like perfume to you. You will take a whiff, enjoy the smell, and sit down with the person eating it with no problems whatsoever. Why? Because you will be sabotage free. Freedom has no cravings.

PRESENT MOMENT

Living in the present moment is greatly overlooked but is truly important. Certainly when you're in a taxi, you would like the driver to concentrate on the road, right? If you're kissing someone, you'd like him or her to be concentrating on you, right? When the dentist is working on your teeth, you would like his/her attention on your mouth, right? This is the present moment.

A great way to practice this method is in the shower. Often our minds stray. Who the heck thinks of the present moment when they're in the shower? Not many. Most are thinking about the rest of the day and daydreaming about something else. But if you bring your mind back to the present and enjoy the water, the soap, and the experience, you will eventually get the hang of it. This practice makes meals much better too. Giving gratitude to the food and enjoying every bite. Turn the TV off, put your phone down, stop reading the paper, and just enjoy the food. Stay in the present moment. No past, no future, just peace.

"If you are depressed, you live in the past. If you are anxious, you live in the future. If you are at peace, you live in the present." - Lao Tzu

VISUALIZATION

Visualization is a big part of thinking. Many call this "The Law of Attraction." It's about manifesting your thoughts into reality. You see, energy flows where your focus is. So, if you're focused on the negative, you will continue to attract the negative.

A visualization exercise is very affective. Similar to meditation, you get in position as if you were going to meditate, and envision what it is that you want. But you have to dig deep and actually manifest the feeling.

Example: If your car is on its last leg and you really need a new one, then visualize buying a new car. Imagine signing the papers and driving off the car lot and playing your first song on the radio. Visualize the feelings you would feel and use your driver (mind) to manipulate your horses (emotions). Feel the emotions of it. Keep doing it. Make it a practice. I like to do this exercise right before meditation. Again, putting it out to the universe, then silencing the mind to hear the whispers of the master.

"Therefore I tell you, whatever you ask for in prayer, believe that you have received it, and it will be yours." - Jesus

Doing visualization before meditation is like warming up before working out.

LANGUAGE

In daily life, it's important to switch your perspective and view the glass half full. Instead of saying, "I don't want it to rain" maybe you can say, "I would love for it to be sunny." When something not so great happens in life, find the lesson and seek the opportunity, for improvement is your purpose in life. Everything that happens presents an opportunity. Find it.

Language can play a factor. Look at the word "hate." We often use that word as slang. "I hate mosquitos," "I hate mustard," "I hate when someone cuts me off on the road." Try taking that word out of your language. It's OK to dislike, but not to hate. Not only that, but we are training our children to use the same word. That's not the only word though.

How about swearing? Well, same thing really. Have you ever met someone that can't stop swearing? I mean, every sentence it's an "f bomb" or some other four-letter word? I know they're just words, but they have negative connotations, and in my opinion, it makes you look like you have no vocabulary.

When I discovered this, I took swearing out of my vocabulary. I wanted to try it as an experiment to train my mind. I ended up loving the challenge of it and continued it. A one month experiment then became a new habit. Three years later, I don't swear and don't even think about it. Now don't get me wrong: If I stub my toe, I'm going to say something like "darn it" or "oh my goodness." So again, the reaction is still there, which means the same as a curse word. But man, is it a great mind trainer. I challenge you to try it for a month. You may just like it.

It's funny nobody in my circle ever notices that I don't swear anymore. All that mind training, and the only reward is from within. But isn't that how it's supposed to be?

SOCIAL MEDIA ASSIGNMENT:

Post about your no swearing challenge for thirty days. Spread this awareness to your audience and inspire someone today. I want to know how you're doing.

TAGS: #NoSwearingChallenge #ThreeDLife #EatTheSunlight

HOPE

Hope is so powerful. If you study a survivalist, you will find out just how necessary it is! If one were lost in the wilderness or stuck on a lifeboat in the ocean, hope can never be lost. As soon as hope is lost, in most cases, you will die. Hope is what keeps us alive and helps motivate us through the toughest challenges.

This plays a factor in health as well. In Bernie Siegel MD's book, *Love, Medicine and Miracles*, he often tells stories of his patients getting better with hope!

He speaks of patients who were given "fake medicine" and told it would make them better. The "fake medicine" played no factor in healing them, but yet they did. The "fake medicine" gave these people hope and helped de-stress them, which in turn opened lymphatic and emotional obstructions.

Siegel also speaks of many situations where a cancer patient will quit his or her job and start taking part in activities that he or she always wanted to do (or already truly enjoys). Some patients travel the world, go skydiving, or spend more time with their loved ones. Many of these patients lived a few more decades when they were only given a few more months. You see, by changing their lives, they de-stressed, and every month or year that went by, they developed more hope.

There are many studies done where people get the same diseases as their parents and die around the same age. They feel they are doomed. This lack of hope usually results in them being destructive and leads to food and substance abuse.

Mickey Mantle is an excellent example of this. His family had a history of dying young from Hodgkin's. The baseball icon thought he would die by age forty, so he smoke, drank, and partied on a legendary level. He ended up living to sixty-three, but suffered in poor health. In 1995, he became the most famous person to ever to need a liver transplant. Unfortunately, two of his sons developed the same fear and hopelessness as they became substance abusers and died at the ages of thirty-six and forty-seven.

"If I knew I was going to live this long. I would have taken better care of myself."
- Mickey Mantle

Bottom line: No hope brings forth a limited chance of survival because of the physical and mental obstructions.

SELF-CARE

The average person is too busy in life and in their mind to practice self-care. Self-care is a great way to feel good about ourselves, pamper ourselves, and most importantly, have fun! What is life without fun?

Hobbies

Self-care starts directly with hobbies. Hobbies provide a slice of work-free and responsibility-free time in your schedule. This can be especially welcome for people who feel overwhelmed by all that they have to do, and need to recharge their batteries by doing something they enjoy. For those who feel overwhelmed by responsibility, it may be difficult to find the time or give themselves permission to take a break from a busy schedule and just sit and relax.

Engaging in hobbies can provide a break with a purpose, which can help people feel that they're not just 'sitting around,' but are using their down time for something productive. Either way, hobbies provide a nice break in a busy week.

I used to be one of those people who only concentrated on work. I've lost relationships because of it, and I've lost touch with family members because of it. I now understand the value and have made hobbies a part of my life.

Using myself as an example, I love going to the movies. It's a great way to escape for a few hours, and I have no problem going by myself in the middle of the day. Of course, years ago, it was a problem because of my food addiction, but I had to overcome that. I enjoy going to local events that include meeting like-minded people. I use Meetup.com as a resource for that. And for my drama, I follow the WWE (they're my action-packed soap operas), and every now and again, I'll start a new series on Netflix and binge out. But perhaps my favorite hobby is finding a peaceful place, usually with water, and enjoying some alone time visualizing and meditating outside.

I'd like you to pause for the cause right now and write down your top five favorite hobbies. And next to them, put why you like them, and the last time you did them. If you don't like what you see, it's time to step up your game. Hobbies are important. You must have fun!

Me-Day

The "me-day" is something I learned a few years back. It simply means taking a day for yourself. Turn the phone off, unplug from the digital world, and date yourself!

Example: Ladies can go get their hair and nails done, then go to their favorite lunch spot, see a movie, and then enjoy a fun hobby. And most importantly, do it by yourself. That's the trick. One must spend time with themselves to get to know one's self.

Our schedules are packed with responsibilities and activities for others. Without scheduling time for ourselves, we will continuously wait for a time when things are less hectic or when we have achieved all of our goals. That time may never come. So plan a me-day ahead of time and put it in your schedule. Drop the kids off at a trusted family member's home and take some time to do whatever you want to.

I recommend performing a "me-day" once per month.

SOCIAL MEDIA ASSIGNMENT:

Post about your me-day. Spread this awareness to your audience and inspire someone today. What did you do on your day? Movies? Massage? Lunch? Did you turn your phone off?

Tell me about your great day and how you felt about it.

TAGS: #MeDay #ThreeDLife #EatTheSunlight #DeStress

SIMPLE PLEASURES

Simple pleasures is a game I play with clients. It simply includes recognizing something simple in everyday life that brings you a good feeling. They happen everyday; we just need to have gratitude for them happening. Here is a list of some examples:

1. Sleeping in on a rainy day: As the rain beats lightly against the window, you nestle your head deeper into your pillow. The sound is soothing and your bed feels like a sanctuary. There is no place you would rather be.

2. Finding money you didn't know you had: You reach into your pocket and find a twenty dollars from the last time you wore these jeans. You aren't rich, but you are richer than you were a second earlier.

3. Making brief eye contact with someone you're attracted to: You pass her or him on the street or in the subway. They glance up at you momentarily, making direct eye contact in a way that seems to communicate a subtle curiosity. For a split second, it makes you think…and then it's gone.

4. Making the yellow light: It's one of the most common simple pleasures—the act of beating the pack. As you blaze through the yellow light, you glance in your rearview to see all the cars behind you stopping at the red light. Yes! You made it!

5. Hearing the right song at the right moment: It doesn't matter what the setting is, hearing the right song is one of those simple pleasures that instantly lifts your spirits. You could be driving home from work, hanging out at a bar with friends, or jogging. When the right song rattles your eardrums, the entire meaning of life seems crystal clear.

6. The first sip of a beverage when you're thirsty: You just finished mowing the lawn or taking a long jog. The only thing on your mind is an ice-cold glass of water. When you are really, really thirsty, that first sip of any liquid beverage is sheer bliss.

SOCIAL MEDIA ASSIGNMENT:

Post your simple pleasures as they happen to you. Spread this awareness to your audience and inspire someone today.

TAGS: #SimplePleasure #ThreeDLife #EatTheSunlight #DeStress

YOUR WORK

The system is set up so that you need money to support yourself. But what you do for work is up to you in most cases. Your job or career can play a pivotal role in your happiness, for everyone wants to do what they love.

I know many people who have jobs they strongly dislike. If you are one of these people, then I say to you, start looking for another job. It's just not worth it in my opinion. There are other jobs out there you can get.

I know many people who love what they do! They get up everyday and are excited to go to work. If you are one of those people, then I say to you, congratulations.

I know many entrepreneurs. Entrepreneurs are some of the most happily stressed people in the world. They love what they do, but their competitive ego always wants to build and grow, so they are always plotting and planning. If you are one of these people, then I say to you, just be careful and make sure to take breaks.

And then you have service people. These are people who don't care about the money and don't need to, as they are unplugged from the system. I stay at an Ashram yearly, so I'm familiar with this way of life. When you live at an Ashram, you become part of a community. Your job is to contribute in a communal form. You may work the kitchen, you may perform maintenance duties, you may do house cleaning, or you may work in the garden. You receive a room and food, and you provide a purpose to your community. These are some of the happiest people I have ever met. Money plays no factor.

The Eightfold Path in Buddhism is a great lifestyle blueprint and one of the eight principles is called "Right Livelihood." It simply means doing work that is right. If you work a job that is against your values, then you will internally suffer as your master will cry. Example: If you don't eat flesh and are passionate about animal rights, then working for a burger joint would be wrong for you. So if you are working at a job that messes with your consciousness, get out.

If you're single and have no children, then you have more room to choose the right job or career. If you have children, then your kids are your most important priority, so it's easy to get caught in a job you don't like to pay the bills. Be patient, use your horse and carriage, and find the correct situation for you. I think it's important to do the right work that suits you. Everyone wants to have purpose.

One time I was in the sauna at the gym and an older guy was dropping gems about working in society. He was a retired accountant and in his early sixties. He said, "If you work your job to make a living, then retire as soon as you can and enjoy the second phase of your life, but if you love your job or you're an entrepreneur who loves the thrill, never stop."

The first person I thought of when he said this was Vince McMahon. Mr. McMahon loves being the CEO of the WWE. He bought the company in the early 1980s and has transformed the WWE into a global juggernaut, completely changing the pro wrestling business. He is currently sixty-nine and will die on his throne because he loves his job! Another person this applies to is Larry King! King is eighty and is still interviewing people. He loves his work! Some others still working and thriving are Al Pacino (seventy-four), Hugh Hefner (eighty-eight), Martha Stewart (seventy-one), Warren Buffett (eighty-three), Oprah Winfrey (sixty), Jack Nicholson (seventy-seven), Dan Rather (eighty-two), Don Rickles (eighty-eight), Clint Eastwood (eighty-four), Chuck Norris (seventy-four), and certainly there are many out there who are not "celebrities." Your work counts.

RELATIONSHIPS

Whether it's our family, friends, or significant other, drama tends to find us. Anytime two humans come together, friction may occur; it's just a part of life. But every relationship brings value and lessons to learn from. Let's get your inner circle in order. Start by making a list of your ten "best" circle members.

One of the keys of a good relationship is letting go of expectations. You can't expect your family member, friend, or significant other to believe or feel what you do. You don't want to expect them to be a certain way. You must accept who they are as they walk their path. No one likes to be criticized or lectured. I do my best to only give advice or opinions when they are called upon. Otherwise, it comes off as judgment.

Being a good circle member consists of:

1. Keeping promises

2. Staying loyal

3. Being respectful

4. Being supportive

5. Being a good listener

6. Being there in time of need

7. Giving thoughtful advice when asked

8. Being forgiving

Sometimes, you have someone in your life that you are very close with, but you hold resentment toward, and you just don't enjoy being around him or her. Maybe they're too negative or they don't have similar interests. You may have known this person your whole life, but when the phone rings and you see their name, you don't feel like picking up. You feel loyalty toward this person, but you know the conversation is going to exhaust you or make you emotional in some way or another. This is not a healthy way to live.

I want you to imagine your inner circle as a closet full of clothes. Each piece of clothing is a person in your circle. And just like clothes, some shirts you wear often, and some occasionally. The ones you wear often can come to the front for easy access and the occasional can go toward the back. This is a great way to manage your relationships. The people you enjoy associating with come to the front and the people who are occasional should go to the back. The problem is, the people who should be occasional are often engaged with too consistently. You have to decide who you want to be consistent with and who you want to be occasional with. Take some time and look at your top ten list. In the name of your health, which ones should be consistent and which ones should be occasional?

Now start putting space in between your occasional circle members. Don't talk or see them weekly, talk or see them monthly, or even quarterly. Sure, they may realize it after some time and make mention of it. And when that happens, remember you're dealing with the ego part of the mind. Be gentle, yet honest, and remember, it's your life and you're in control.

RESENTMENT

You know the feeling. Having someone in your inner circle who has consistently done something or hasn't done something for you over a period of time. This feeling is called resentment. When you resent someone, it leads to hypersensitivity, which means this person could do the slightest thing to rub you the wrong way, and you will react dramatically.

"Anger will never disappear so long as thoughts of resentment are cherished in the mind. Anger will disappear just as soon as thoughts of resentment are forgotten." - John Dryden

Perhaps you resent a parent because he or she never gave you the love you felt you deserved. Or you resent a longtime friend because they always borrow your stuff and never bring it back. Or maybe you resent your significant other because every time you want to go out and have fun, they'd rather sit home and watch TV.

Resentment builds over time and becomes a toxicity that can ruin any relationship. Many married couples resent each other and go many years without addressing it. This is very damaging and unhealthy for the human body.

All that said, it is very difficult to approach the person you resent and express yourself. You are full of fear in doing so. The questions run through your mind (driver). How will they react? Will they walk out on me? Will they just challenge and resist what I'm saying? What if I hurt their feelings?

"Resentment always hurts you more than it does the person you resent. While your offender has probably forgotten the offense and gone on with life, you continue to stew in your pain, perpetuating the past. Those who hurt you in the past cannot continue to hurt you now unless you hold on to the pain through

resentment. Your past is past. Nothing will change it. You are only hurting yourself with your bitterness. For your own sake, learn from it, and then let it go." - Rick Warren

It's important to talk to the person you resent; to make them understand why you feel the way you do. If their ego gets bruised that bad, and they never talk to you again, perhaps it is for the better. Love conquers all, and if this person really loves you, they will apologize, explain themselves, and even look for a solution.

THE RESENTMENT LETTER ASSIGNMENT

Write a letter to someone in your life who gets under your skin and makes you emotional. You may carry feelings such as blame, anger, and shame toward this individual. Be honest with your feelings and let it all out. Write this letter as though you will NOT be giving it to your selected person. Do not hold anything back!

The Letter Process:

1. I am writing you this letter because (give your reasons)...

2. Write a paragraph for each reason with more detail.

3. Close your letter with a "wrap-up" or conclusion of what you think can be done to solve these issues.

Don't be surprised if you shed some tears while writing. I have clients cry all the time on this assignment. When you're done with your letter, you will be surprised as to how much better you feel and how much clearer you are on your emotions. Perhaps now you will be ready to give this letter to the person you resent, or at least talk to them about it. Or, maybe you don't. Either way, I recommend you write the letter.

SOCIAL MEDIA ASSIGNMENT:

Post about the experience of writing your resentment letter. Did you cry? Did you get emotional? Did you feel it helped you? Tell me about it.

TAGS: #ResentmentLetter #ThreeDLife #EatTheSunlight #DeStress

---

GRATITUDE & LOVE

Certainly we've all said "thank you" to somebody in our lives. Perhaps it was when someone held the door open for you, or someone passed the salt at the dinner table, or a friend did a favor for you. But gratitude is bigger than just saying "thank you." Gratitude is an empowering feeling that borders the emotion love. It's an appreciation for people, places, things, actions, and nature.

Have you ever been so grateful that you feel a tingly feeling overcome your body? That's energy at work. It's actually very similar to love. Love is expressed as an action and experienced as a feeling.

"Gratitude teaches us to appreciate the rainbow, and the storm."
- Christina G. Hibbert, PsyD

We often throw the word "love" around like it was nothing. How many times do you use the word "love" in your language? "Oh I love that restaurant. I love that television show. I love cheddar cheese." And how nervous or excited are we when we're in a new relationship and the "L word" is used for the first time! Do you call your best friend right away and start the convo like this…"Guess what he or she said?"

But you see, love isn't just a 'throw-around' word in our language, and love isn't just for romance—it's for all. Love is not killing that spider that you find crawling on your wall. Love is not hating another person, even if they harmed you or your family. Love is forgiving someone who has wronged you. Love is not judging another person no matter what they have done. Love is helping a homeless person or a stray animal. Love is compassion, and most importantly, love is the universal religion of mankind.

There is a famous saying that goes:

"Buddha was not a Buddhist. Jesus was not a Christian. Muhammad was not a Muslim. They were teachers who taught love. Love was their religion."

Gratitude is the way we appreciate and celebrate our love. It's waking up in the morning and being thankful for another day. It's being thankful for another meal before you eat. It's going outside and feeling thankful for nature. It's contacting a friend or family member just to say "I appreciate you and all you have done for me." It's even finding a lesson within a horrible experience that has happened in your life. Sometimes it's looking at the glass half full. It's the expression, acknowledgment, and thankfulness of love and lessons.

If you have ever been called "ungrateful" in recent memory, then maybe you have some work to do. Being ungrateful can be a symptom of a negative toxicity that is growing inside of you. This toxicity goes hand-and-hand with the negative thinking we spoke about earlier and can manifest into poor health. Having gratitude for all that happens can release the tension and stress that comes from life. Start today.

SOCIAL MEDIA ASSIGNMENT:

Tag one or more people that you have gratitude for, and publicly show your appreciation. Tell them how much they mean to you and that you are there for them. This random expression will ignite a warm feeling that will jolt through their body.

TAGS: #Gratitude #ThreeDLife #EatTheSunlight

THE GRATITUDE LETTER ASSIGNMENT

Write a gratitude letter to the same person you wrote your resentment letter to! Be honest with your feelings and let it all out. Write this letter as though you will NOT be giving it to your selected person. Do not hold anything back!

The Letter Process:

1. I am writing you this letter because I am grateful for (give your reasons)...

2. Write a paragraph for each reason with more detail.

3. Close your letter with a "wrap-up" or conclusion of your expression

Don't be surprised if you shed some tears while writing. I have clients cry all the time on this assignment. When you're done with your letter, you will be surprised as to how much better you feel and how much clearer you are on your emotions. Perhaps now you will be ready to give this letter to the person you resent and appreciate, or at least talk to them about it. Or, maybe you don't. Either way, I recommend you write the letter.

SOCIAL MEDIA ASSIGNMENT:

Post about the experience of writing your gratitude letter. Did you cry? Did you get emotional? Did you feel it helped you? Tell me about it.

TAGS: #GratitudeLetter #ThreeDLife #EatTheSunlight #DeStress

#ThreeDLife
Success Stories

I started as a damaged, defeated, and toxic person whose hair was falling out. I lived off of soda and cigarettes and thought the world revolved around me! But Kevin has such a unique teaching style, and it makes it hard not to listen. Although I resisted at first, I started to understand the teachings and began applying them to my life. I stopped drinking soda. I stopped smoking. I lost weight. And my hair is growing back! I think I'm more patient and more conscious of my thoughts. My whole life I've always sabotaged myself, but now I get rid of those thoughts before the actions come. I handle a lot of situations differently. The biggest thing that I've learned from the program is that gratitude changes everything! They used to tell me I was "ungrateful." And now I'm grateful for everything. I look for the lesson in everything that happens. I feel different and look at things differently. I think I have more work to do, but I know I can live this #ThreeDLife.

-Natasha Threet

ACCEPTANCE

Life happens, and situations that seem negative to you will happen. There is nothing you can do about that. People will die, possessions will be stolen, and you won't get along with everyone. Can you accept this?

I remember reaching out to my spiritual teacher because someone had "stabbed me in the back" in my life. I was very hurt and upset. He taught me that it's normal to be "wronged." This concept hit home. It made sense to me right away. We don't live in a glass bubble, and certainly every human doesn't live by the same rules or codes that you do.

A friend of mine was recently "wronged" by a man she was dating for over a year. Come to find out, he was not only seeing another woman, but was engaged! My friend was crushed, and like many "scorned" people, she sought revenge as rage filled her soul. She justified it as "doing the right thing" because she felt that the girl he was going to marry should know who she was marrying. But I informed her that every action has a reaction, and the reaction coming back on her may not be pretty. I let her know that she's supposed to be wronged by another human, for it's part of her journey. It's what will make her grow, and believe it or not, it's part of what will make him grow too.

Last summer I was enjoying a mountain bike I had bought myself. I hadn't ridden a bike since I was a kid, and I was having a great time making ten-mile rides all over the surrounding towns. And then one morning, the bike was gone. Someone had stolen it right off the property. I was amazed as to how much it didn't bother me. It took me only a few minutes to accept it and understand that it was gone and there was nothing I could do about it.

Acceptance can also be used with your inner circle. Perhaps you have a significant other or friend who does something that annoys you. If you do not accept this "bad habit," then it can turn to resentment. Accept people for who they are and how they act, for you can't go trying to change everyone.

So accept that your car might break down or get dented. Accept that someone you know may "wrong" you. Accept that it rains. Accept that there will be traffic on the highway sometimes. Accept that you will be taxed. Accept that you will need to invest money into the house you own. Accept that the pet you love so much will die. Accept that "circumstance" will happen, so when it does happen, you can take away the lessons without being scorned.

THE LIBRARY

I'm sure you weren't expecting a section on this subject.

There was a time in my life where things were rough, and the library was my place of refuge. The environment helped me get work done, and it helped me know myself better. I still to this day spend a lot of time at the library and highly encourage you to too.

It's a friendly and quiet place where you can get work done, use their resources, or just simply relax. If you want to get away from the hustle and bustle of your life, pack a lunch and head off to library land. Find a nice corner and read, visualize, or meditate. Relax, enjoy the solitude, and be alone with yourself. I look at each library as a mini Ashram.

PICK-ME-UPS

Every now and again, the untrained human mind creates sadness. But you don't have to be sad. And you certainly don't need food to comfort you! Here are a few ways you can give yourself a pick-me-up:

1. Listen to music

2. Bounce

3. Make High-Pitched Noises

Listening to music is great! Pick the kind that amps you up, puts you in your zone, or relaxes you. Your mood will change. Perhaps it's while you're driving or maybe it's in your living room. There is nothing wrong with putting music on and dancing around and visualizing all sorts of things. It helps the mind.

Bouncing is something you probably didn't think of, but boy does it help. You can do it with music or without; all you have to is stand up and start bouncing. You can bounce in place or bounce all over the room or yard. It's great exercise and it gets your body moving. It actually helps move your lymph fluid too. That's an added bonus. If you like it, go get a trampoline! It feels great!

OK, so maybe I'm a weirdo…but that's OK! I'll be the weirdo making high-pitched noises because it changes your mood. It certainly doesn't require any work. Just make sure no one is around, and start belting out high-pitched noises. You can do short ones, or long ones. This method works like a charm. This is why so many people live longer who own pets, because they perform "baby talk" to their cats or dogs. It feels good. Make some noises right now!

FITNESS

Being "in shape" does not make you healthy! Humans are getting sicker and sicker and that does not exclude people who work out on a regular basis. The gym cannot save you from years of toxic waste congestion and inflammation. In fact, the more muscles you have, the more places acids have to absorb and hide.

However, fitness does play a part in having health and vitality. In order to keep the body strong, one must exercise. The muscles, the tendons, and the ligaments must all be worked. And most importantly, the heart! Obviously, fitness is popular and you have tons of fitness gurus out there preaching their different ways of doing things, but in this book, I tell you to keep it natural!

Cardio

A good cardio routine is a must for any human. Getting the heart pumping and blood flowing is essential for a healthy body. I feel that cardio should be the core and foundation of your fitness routine.

In my opinion, the best cardio one can do is running. I honestly don't understand the elliptical machines. If someone were chasing you, you wouldn't "elliptical" down the street! Yes, I know some people talk about their knees or feet hurting. But that's because of acids in most cases. So, if you eat the sunlight and go by the #ThreeDLife, those acids can be cleaned out and you can get back to running again! It's natural and humans are meant to run!

Weight Training

I enjoy weight training. It's challenging and certainly builds muscle if you're doing it correctly.

However, it can be considered unnatural. Some of these machines are giving humans a lane to get super buffed up. I'm pretty sure in caveman times, there were no humans resembling the Incredible Hulk!

Another thing about weight training is that it usually makes humans aggressive! And to make matters worse, weight training adds trauma to the body.

If you're going to do weight training, stick to free weights and keep it simple: squats, deadlifts, curls, military press, etc.

High Intensity Interval Training

I respect HIIT! It's so challenging and so effective. You perform short bursts of intense bodyweight exercises (pushups, burpees, crunches, etc.) and cardio exercises (jumping jacks, mountain sprints, high-knees), then take a short break, then go again. It's an amazing way to burn fat, stay fit, and give your body a chance to be naturally strong and fast. Isn't that what we really want? To be able to run, jump, push, and pull? Survival of the fittest!

We created a HIIT routine that can work for you. I call it the thirty-ten fitness routine. It consist of an exercise that's thirty seconds followed by one that is ten seconds.

Here is a quick break down:

30 Jumping jacks

10 Squats

30 Upward mountain climbers

10 Floor jumps

BREAK (60 seconds)

30 Floor sprint climbers

10 Push-ups

30 Ab Bicycles

10 Spiderman planks

BREAK (60 seconds)

Now repeat this three times and you have yourself a great twenty minute workout that you can do anywhere anytime with NO equipment!

HIIT to me is a test. It truly gives a measure as to how in shape your body is. A lot of the weight training guys can't do HIIT. That's because they're not in shape—they're just strong.

We have this fitness routine on video and provide it to our clients that do our #ThreeDLife *12-Week Jump Start*.

Yoga

Yoga can be defined as an ascetic discipline, which includes breath control, simple meditation, and the adoption of specific bodily postures. Yoga is widely practiced for health and relaxation. Derived from India, yoga has been used for centuries, yet is just now becoming widely popular in America.

The first thing I think about with yoga is how challenging it is! Some people have trouble with it because they're not flexible (myself included) and their minds have trouble slowing down to a yoga pace. I fit this description certainly, and I struggle with it, especially when I first started.

However, I must be as honest as possible. I believe there is no other exercise or method better suited for the human body. Think about it: You get to strengthen your muscles, stretch your muscles, move your lymph, break a sweat, master the obstacles of the mind, all while not putting ANY major trauma on your body!

Here are some benefits of a yoga practice:

1. Back pain treatment

2. Fertility aid

3. Helps with heart issues

4. Helps with lung issues

5. Helps with arthritis and fibromyalgia

6. Helps with insomnia

7. Helps with MS

8. Helps the mind focus

9. Great de-stressor

10. Moves lymph

11. Strengthens muscles

12. Stretches your muscles, ligaments, and tendons

If you had a yoga practice, you would build great muscle and become more flexible. Weight training is not necessary to get fit and have lean muscle.

I recommend incorporating a yoga practice into your fitness routine. I have clients start with a ten-minute routine in the morning and then work up to thirty minutes. Eventually, you want to get up to over an hour. You should try different styles at home on DVD or online, and when you're ready, try out some live classes at a yoga studio. I think at least three to five days a week is fantastic.

Your Exercise Routine

To make your exercise routine complete, I think you should use running as your foundation and then supplement it with yoga and or HIIT. If you're dead set on weight training, then mix it in too, but don't slack on the cardio.

All and all, I like the combo of HIIT, yoga, and running best.

If you're an obese person, I do not recommend exercise outside of yoga, swimming, or walking. You need to detoxify your body before doing heavy exercise, or the acids and waste will just go back into circulation due to congested lymph (your sanitation department), poor kidney function (cellular waste exit), and poor bowel function (digestive waste exit). This can cause injuries and certainly bring forth an acute situation such as stroke, heart attack, or an asthma attack.

Just recently, I saw that an obese man died who was doing one of those protein powder MLM schemes. The poor guy was trying to change his life around and was desperate for help. Of course one of those "promoters" who is into fitness led him down the path of protein powders and heavy activity in the gym. Remember, there are only two ways we feel physical pain, and that's trauma and acids. So what this desperate guy was doing was consuming more acids in an already very acidic body. All while the workout was causing trauma and releasing more stored wastes and acids from his tissues. This is a formula for disaster.

I urge you, if you're obese, please stop focusing on weight loss and a high protein diet! Start thinking about a full natural lifestyle change and meet with a natural health professional who can coach you. The weight loss will come as a side effect of healing yourself, and you will be able to build muscle later. Have patience and enjoy the journey. Eventually you will inspire others.

SOCIAL MEDIA ASSIGNMENT:

Post about your fitness routines. Are you doing yoga? Are you running? Are you doing our thirty-ten HIIT workout? Tell me about it.

TAGS: #Yoga or #HIIT or #Cardio #ThreeDLife #EatTheSunlight #DeStress

---

MORNING ROUTINE

The first thing I do when working with a client is put them on a morning routine. Being in a morning routine sets the pace of the day and has worked wonders with my clients. Here is the morning routine I recommend you perform every day:

1. As soon as you wake up, get on the floor with your back against the bed

2. Visualize or pray

3. Perform meditation for five minutes (or longer)

2. Chug sixteen ounces of room temperature spring water

3. Perform a ten-minute yoga routine (or longer)

4. Make and drink your Sunlight Smoothie

SOCIAL MEDIA ASSIGNMENT:

Post about your morning routine. Is it helping? Did it set your day off right? How do you feel when you skip it?

TAGS: #MorningRoutine #ThreeDLife #EatTheSunlight #DeStress

WHAT NOW?

It's time to put it all together! Handle your resentment issues, practice self-care, have like-minded people around you, make a living doing something enjoyable, think and speak positive, get quality sleep, practice your morning routine, and of course, always have the awareness of your horse and carriage!

If you want to live the #ThreeDLife, then keep practicing so that stress doesn't pierce your new SUNLIGHT shield! Remember, real stress is fight or flight in an emergency situation. But external drama? It's all up to your driver (mind). So next time someone or something stresses you out or causes a certain emotion, tell yourself, "This isn't stress; I'm not being chased by a lion!"

Let's bring this mind-induced stress way down, so your physical body (carriage) can thrive without any physical or mental obstructions. Mental obstructions can cause physical obstructions.

INTERVIEW WITH A MYSTIC

During my transformational journey, I met Nashid Fareed-Ma'at while staying at an Ashram in the mountains. Upon meeting him, I sensed the warmth of his heart and began asking a slew of questions as I desired to learn more. He was and still is kind enough to pass on what he has learned.

On his mystical path of the heart, Nashid has been influenced by a number of spiritual traditions, including Kemetic spirituality, Sufism, and Islam, Buddhism, Christianity, and Yoga-Vedanta. This path has also led him into the art of writing, particularly poetry, and West African drumming.

Nashid is the most committed and knowledgeable spiritual individual I have ever met, and I thought it would be of value to interview him and pass the recording exclusively to my clients. When I began writing this project, it was a no brainer to transcribe parts of that recording and share them with you. He has contributed to my growth greatly, and I hope that can spread to you.

KWR: One of the things I teach and encourage clients to do is meditation. In your opinion, what is the importance of meditation?

Nashid: For someone like myself whose spiritual practice is my main focus in my life, it's the foundation. It's the foundation to living a life that's in alignment with truth and love. The meditation allows us to have space where that can be and deepens the realization of having a peaceful life. Most of us are so focused on the ways of the world and the conditions we find ourselves in, we tend to think outside of ourselves, and we lose focus to that which is within us. And within us is a means to have a life that's peaceful. Meditation is essential for at least the approach that I take, which is guided by the spiritual teachings specifically of a mystic nature. Meditation is the foundation that allows that house to be built.

KWR: Do you think morning is the best time to put meditation into your routine?

Nashid: Many traditions that I have studied point to the morning. In fact, many point to the time the sun rises or right after the sun rises, as a time to have a point of focus. I also acknowledge that many of us are transitioning into a meditative practice. I try to take the easier approach. For example, a morning person may have an easier time establishing a practice in the morning. If you're a night person, make time at night. If you're a midday person, make time to do it at that time. More so to establish the practice. I think once the person sees the benefits of the practice, then it may be time to make certain changes that will require discipline and adjustments. But for establishing a practice, it's better to have a regular time, so I suggest not fluctuating times. So if you're going to get up at 7:00 a.m. and meditate for fifteen minutes, do that everyday at that time. If you're a night person, maybe you do it at 7:00 p.m. and just be consistent with that. And the practice will start to grow.

KWR: What do you say to someone who has struggled with his or her mind being too active and wandering during meditation? Even after a month or so of practicing?

Nashid: Patience. The mind is a creature of conditioning. Look at a baby; their minds are not usually as active as adults, but if they are around adults with active minds, then they will become conditioned to have an active mind. The natural state of the mind is to be in a state of relaxation, so the mind can observe, and we can navigate through the world. We are conditioned to use the mind in other ways, and we learn to have our minds be overly active. We use the mind to make decisions, which is actually not the purpose of the mind. Whatever your situation is that brings you to the meditative practice, whatever challenges you encounter, be patient. If you looked at your life on a film screen and saw all the things that played into the conditioning of the mind, you would see many years of it. We can't expect our minds to be conditioned to be relaxed in a month or so. It's not a healthy approach. One of the things a meditative practice allows to happen is that it gives us a mirror to see how our mind is operating. For so many people, their minds are overly active, and they're not even aware that they're operating in an overly active manner. Just to come to that realization, that's a benefit; it's part of the journey of establishing a meditative practice. So be patient. But also, let's look at location. You want to be in a quiet room so the mind doesn't become distracted. Posture is important. You want to sit upright to allow the body to relax. The mind and body are like best friends, so if the body is relaxed, it will encourage the mind to be relaxed. And breathing is important. We can breathe in a way to bring things more to a center, allowing the mind and body to relax. This can help pull the overactive mind back and allow it to rest in its natural state.

KWR: And as we get deeper into our meditative practice, do you feel that we can now control the mind in everyday life?

Nashid: I avoid the word "control" because I think we usually put ourselves in less of a position of control when we try to control the mind. The things that we try to control with the mind are the thoughts, so if you try to control the mind with another thought, you're actually adding another thought to a series of thoughts that are usually out of control. So you're contributing to the dynamic of being further out of control. I prefer the word restraint, so that we can understand that the mind may be conditioned in a certain way. It's something that keeps us in this uncontrollable flow of the mind. When that tendency of the mind arises, we want to acknowledge it because we don't want to cover it up. We have the ability that once there's a suggestion or tendency of the mind in the forefront of our consciousness, we can turn our focus elsewhere. I've been taught the breath. So if there is a thought in my mind that is not helpful meditatively or in life in general, at any point, through my practice, I can turn my attention from that thought to my breath, let the thought pass, let the mind become more quiet to see what's going on, and then merely observe. And then when I have a better idea of what's happening, I can make a decision. When we establish a meditative practice, it allows us to see that there is the mind, but there is something beyond the mind that's observing the mind. As much as the mind can make suggestions, we don't have to follow the suggestions. There is a place of discernment, and there starts to be this space that's created between the mind and that for which I truly am, which observes the mind. It's easier to realize the dynamic while meditating, but when it becomes a daily practice we start to be able to do that in everyday life. So instead of having just a meditative practice, our lives become meditative. This changes the dynamic of how one deals with life.

KWR: And of course, this plays a major factor in how we deal with stress.

Nashid: Yeah. The things we say stress us out really don't stress us out. It's our mind. It's how we react to the stressors. That's not to say there are not things in life that aren't stressful. There are stressful things in life by all means, and it's natural to feel some type of stress because we are dealing with a stressful situation. It's like walking into a hot room and feeling warm. If you don't feel warm, that's more of a concern. But there is a difference between walking into the hot room and getting totally pulled into doing things that are beyond control because you're reacting to the heat. And walking into the same room and being centered within yourself. Now you can make a decision and not be pulled into a reaction or pulled into doing things. If you can quiet the mind to hear the whispers of the heart, you will always know what to do.

KWR: How important is it to live in the present moment?

Nashid: People will come to that realization themselves in a daily meditative practice that the most peaceful way to live is by living in the moment. If you start to dissect your problems, you will find they are tied to the past in some way; that we have allowed the past to intrude on the present, whether we're dealing with things that are happening now by looking through the lens of the past (which blinds ourselves from being happy now). A lesser percentage is tied to the future, but even the future we tend to project from the past. It's not like we project to the future with a clean slate; it's usually based on what our past was. If it was fulfilling, then we want more. It kind of keeps us in bondage, in the sense that there are so many opportunities in the present to make life better, but we lose sight of those opportunities a lot of times when our means of perceiving the present are so conditioned by the past.

KWR: With practicing these ways, do you feel one could go through life with no emotional pain or not as much emotional pain?

Nashid: It's not to say that you won't have painful experiences. But there is a difference between going through a painful experience and having the experience define your life. If you have a mind and body in this world, there are going to be unfortunate things that happen; it's part of life. But there is a way to move through these experiences without them scaring us or defining us. It's not so much that the suffering hurts us—it's how we interact with the suffering and a lot of times, it's the reaction. That's the conditioning of the mind. Let's say one's father passes away. If one were to have a good relationship with his or her father, he or she is going to be sad and in mourning. But when you have a meditative practice, it allows a person to observe the mind and it now gives you a choice to go with the sadness of the mind or go with a deliberative peaceful approach. So now you don't have to follow the suggestion of the mind. The meditative practice allows us to come to a genuine realization of these things in play.

CHAPTER 5

DETOX

WHAT IS DETOX?

Detox, in simple terms, is the removal of toxic substances from a living organism. In our case, the human body. It is considered by me and my colleagues as a process used as a tool to help someone heal versus a "quick fix" like the "establishment's" pills and procedures. It has become a trend in modern times, which has made it a buzzword that people enjoy throwing around. But most have no idea what it truly is and most have never truly practiced the process.

A toxin, as it relates to a health detox, is an antigenic, usually of a foreign poison or of a waste product origin. The reality is that no matter how healthy you live or think you live, toxins will enter your body through your foods, drinks, hygiene products, and air. And if that's not enough, we have leftover wastes that a congested lymphatic system wasn't able to remove. It's important to the home you call a body, to clean out. After all, when you have a party at your house, don't you clean up after?

These toxins float through your blood or lymph and eventually find a home stored inside tissues. Tissues make up glands, organs, muscle, and skin. If you're overweight, toxins can be stored in your extra fat, and if you're in shape, toxins can be stored in your extra muscle. Of course the longer they're stored, the more damage they do to your cells, as toxins are on the acidic side of chemistry. And what do acids do? They burn. And what does burning do? It inflames.

If you want to remove toxins, you have to first stop ingesting food that promotes acids and mucus. This means one must go on a strict diet that consists of no protein, starch, or artificial foods. Secondly, you want to decongest lymph fluid (your sanitation department) and get it moving to bring these toxins to your exits.

And thirdly, you want to have your exits open, so these toxins can be removed to the outside world.

We need our two main exits to be open and working correctly: the kidneys (cellular waste) and the bowels (digestive waste). If your two main exits aren't working correctly, these toxins will only loosen from the tissue, go back into circulation, and eventually find a new home in another clump of tissue.

HAVE YOU DETOXED BEFORE?

I'm assuming you have experienced detox before, because you probably had the flu once or twice in your life. When you get the flu, your body is detoxing. You contracted a virus or bacteria, and now the body is doing its work to clean and heal. So it goes into a "healing crisis." Your thyroid raises your temperature as your body wants to sweat out toxins. You aren't hungry because your digestive system needs a break. And you feel like you got hit by a truck because acids are being removed from your tissues. So every time you get the flu, it's actually a blessing because your body is cleansing! It's the natural mechanism your living organism (body) goes through.

It's actually an opportunity, as the body is purging itself of other flaws you have built up over the years. But we don't usually look at it that way. Getting the flu is an inconvenience to us busy earthlings, so we go get medicines or even worse, flu shot vaccines.

THE THREE PILLARS OF DETOX

Detox can be categorized as either performing a cleanse or a detox intensive. A cleanse is fruit or juice feasting, which can easily be maintained in one's daily life. A detox intensive is a long process with protocols that should be led by a professional coach.

The "third D" of the #ThreeDLife is about removing these toxins from our bodies on a regular basis to promote a clean, well-functioning machine. There are three ways to do so:

1. Fruit Feasting

2. Juice Feasting

3. Botanical Formulas

FRUIT FEASTING

I taught you a lot about fruit in the "diet" section of this book. It's your superhero!

If you wanted to do a simple detox, turn those monkey meals into monkey days! Pick one juicy fruit (oranges, apples, pears, etc.), and eat it all day. The two kinds of fruits that I recommend using are:

1. Grapes (red or purple are strongest)

2. Melons (watermelon is strongest)

These two amazing fruits have power you can't even imagine. They will move your lymph and move it quickly. In fact, if you go on one of these fruits for just five days, you will probably feel like you have a cold. Your nose could start running, and you may sneeze a lot. It's the congested mucus (lymph) starting to break up! One time I did seven monkey days on melons, and I could feel the lymph swishing in my left ear. I have had chronic issues with my left ear for years, and when you start cleansing, you see your weaknesses. Watch out congestion!

While greens are your superhero's sidekick, and support us in daily life, they are not ideal for a detox, unless in juice form. Again, greens, especially leafy greens, are hard to digest and just don't have the same energetic properties as fruit.

That said, if you're ever doing a detox, and things get too intense, you can pump the breaks with greens and salads. The more juicy fruits, the faster you're going to go!

Here is your detox food key:

Juicy Fruit = Gas pedal

Greens = Pumping the brakes

Cooked Greens = Pumping the brakes a little harder

Protein, Fats, or Artificial Foods = Slamming the brakes, causing the airbag to ignite! Dangerous!

SOCIAL MEDIA ASSIGNMENT:

Post about your fruit feast. How do you feel? How is your energy level? Are you noticing progress? Are you doing a mono feast on one kind of fruit? I want to know.

TAGS: #FruitFeast #Detox #MonkeyDay #ThreeDLife #EatTheSunlight

---

JUICE FEASTING

A juice feast is a type of cleanse. I am a big fan of it and do it often. It's a very simple protocol. No solid foods—just all juice.

I spoke about juicing and its benefits earlier in the DIET section of this book, but at this moment, I can tell you to go get a juicer to help with your detox! You can start out with a day or two, and work your way up to a ten-day juice feast. Hopefully, you will work your way up to thirty days.

Many people think they will have low energy during a juice feast, but the opposite is usually the case. When the body is relieved of the task of digesting solid food and given easily absorbable juices instead, an increase in mental and physical energy results. The feeling one gets during a juice feast is exhilarating. People can even go to work during a juice feast, since it supplies all the calories to keep one's energy up. In fact, most people become more productive during the cleanse.

Many people also worry that they will feel hungry during a cleanse. Any feelings of hunger completely disappear after two or three days. I will tell you, the first few days can be hard. Your mind will go through challenges and thoughts you've never had before. You've probably never been hungry before. You thought you were, but it was just your mind tricking you. Now, for the first time in your life, you may have REAL hunger pangs. They will happen in contraction form, maybe every hour or so, for one whole day. Some of you won't get them, and some will. And if and when you do, CONGRATS! It's such an awesome, humbling feeling. I think everyone should feel it. Accept it. And no, don't worry, you're not going to die.

One of the added bonuses of fasting from food is mind training. This goes well with everything I taught you in the DE-STRESS section of this book. Take your mind to the limit, and challenge it. Fasting from solid food will help you beat cravings. It may take a few years of it, but it will. When I did my first juice feasts, I would finish and then eat like a crazy man. Why? Because my cravings were still there. Now, not so much. It just takes time.

I advocate fresh homemade green juice. You simply juice greens and then mix with apples for taste. It's easy! You can add some ginger or turmeric for spice and added benefits. I'm a big fan of adding sprouts as well. I do not recommend a beginner to drink a lot of pure fruit juice. This is because fruit is more powerful than greens, and when you drink all fruit juice, it can bring forth detox symptoms quicker. That said, only drink lots of fruit juice if you're experienced.

Mason jars are highly important in the world of juicing if you're going to be on-the-go. They preserve your juice for the short term. As an added bonus, you can measure out your thirty-two ounces of juice.

THE MASTER CLEANSE

The master cleanse is a famous variation of a juice feast created by Stanley Burroughs in the 1940s. It's a little more intense than a regular juice feast, because instead of juice, you use lemon water with a little bit of maple syrup and cayenne pepper. It's also required that one does a sea salt laxative flush every morning and night. I've done this cleanse twice in my time, and I can assure you it is very effective. The raunchiness that comes out in your bowel movements is immense.

It's generally a ten-day cleanse, but people have been known to go forty days to get a deeper cleaning. What makes this cleanse so intense is the use of lemons. Lemons are extremely astringent and cleansing. That's why they put them in cleaning products.

WATER FASTING

The reason I use the term "feasting" is because someone that water fasts, may take exception to calling it a "juice fast." Fasting is technically not eating or drinking any nutrients outside of the water you drink. I've known people who have water fasted for many days, some up to forty straight, and I can tell you, they would not consider drinking nothing but juice a "fast."

In fact, I performed a seven day "fast" with nothing but herbal teas and water and when I mentioned it to someone who did forty days on water, he made mention of it not being a "fast." I get it, they don't want nothing taken away from there accomplishment. I think we should respect that.

Water fasting is controversial and can be considered dangerous. I do not recommend water fasting more than one day at a time unless you are under the care of a medical doctor or nurse. There are many facilities out there where people can go stay under the watch of a medical staff while fasting.
And even under the care of a medical practitioner, you should ease in properly. You don't want to just go from the standard American diet to a water fast! Now that is extreme! You need to be at a certain level of your detox practice. Experience is key.

In the natural health community, we refer to water fasting as, "mother natures operating table." This is because you can not and should not go forth with your daily life while doing it. It's an at home, stay on the couch type of process and your detox symptoms can and will be intense. Not to mention you will most likely be dizzy. You can hardly walk to the bathroom never mind drive.

If you're reading this book, you are more than likely a beginner at detox. So I recommend trying one day, but nothing beyond that. If you want to learn more, I suggest reading Professor Arnold Ehret's book, *"Rational Fasting."* Professor Ehret is a natural health pioneer and performed a documented forty-nine day water fast in the early 1900's.

BREAKING FAST / FEAST

When doing a juice feast, always ease out of it with raw fruit. The typical rule of thumb is for every three days without solid food, you should eat one day of just fruit. So after a thirty-day juice feast, you should ease out by eating ten days of fruit. After a few days on just fruit, maybe slip some salads in there. But under no circumstance are you to eat starches, protein, or artificial foods. If you do, you can send yourself to the ER. And because the medical establishment doesn't co-sign this level of healing, they will judge it. Now you would be contributing to a reason why they look down on us. Please don't be a reason.

I'm sure you're wondering why coming out of a juice feast eating starches, protein, or artificial foods can send you to the ER. Well, when you're fasting from solid foods, your tubes (vessels and such) tend to constrict. So the foods I just mentioned can get stuck! People have died from breaking a fast with potatoes. Also, your digestive system is on a little vacation, so some of your enzymes that break down food have been resting on the beach catching some sun. You don't want to wake them up with acid and mucus-forming foods! Just don't do it!

While the constricting of your pipes can hurt you if you eat the wrong transitional food, it's a big reason why we call it a "cleanse." When the pipes constrict, it loosens up mucoid matter (plaque) hidden in your tissues. So this "waste" is now being moved out, kind of like squeezing a sponge. This is the advantage of consuming no food. If you were the mayor of a town, and you ordered all city pipes to be cleaned, wouldn't they have to shut down the water first to do so? You must stop the use of the pipes in order to clean them. Certainly your mechanic doesn't give your car an oil change while the engine is running!

And if that isn't enough, how about giving your digestive system a break! Think about this: It takes about eighteen to twenty-four hours for most people before your body eliminates one meal. Considering most of us consume three meals a day full of meat and starches, plus the fact that we love eating processed and packaged foods, your digestive system is working almost all the time! Not only is your digestive system always at work, but you start to build up metabolic waste as all these foods run through you.

Speaking of putting your digestive system on a break: You're going to need to eliminate your bowels to get a successful cleanse. You can do this through the use of enemas.

It is recommended that you perform either an enema or a colon flush at home every two or three days when juice feasting. Enemas are not hard to do, and they are not painful at all. You can bring up a YouTube video to see a tutorial on how to use them. Another option could be drinking a fruit smoothie every few days to bring forth a movement. But enemas are a deeper clean. Remember, what doesn't get eliminated, accumulates.

Here is how you wake up your system on day one of your ease-out:

1. Eat three to five apples or pears

2. A few hours later, have a raspberry and banana smoothie with coconut water

3. A few hours later, have another three to five apples or pears

You can repeat this process on day two of your ease-out if you're not regular yet. You should be back moving your bowels by day three. At that point, you're enzymes are coming back, and you can enjoy the greatness of the other juicy fruit

#ThreeDLife
Success Stories

"I have learned that health is not as complicated as the world makes it seem. I've learned to be more aware of what I put into my body. I have learned to make myself a priority. My diet is completely different, and physically I'm toned from the yoga. A lot of the outbreaks that I was getting on my face are better and that gives me confidence that I'm heading in the right direction."
-Jessica Mays

WHY CLEANSE?

One of the biggest misconceptions is that only fast food junkies are in need of detoxifying their systems. In fact, all bodies can use a cleanse after the heavy load of work it does twenty-four hours a day. Much like you at your job, you need a break. A cleanse provides your digestive system with a quick and easy short-term break. The body knows how to heal; you just have to let it.

Take a few moments to think about the foods and beverages that you consume on a daily basis. Now think about the environment you live and work in, and even the air you breathe. Think about all the medicines you've consumed over the course of your life. There are a lot of toxins that have entered your body. Maybe now is the time to flush lots of those toxins and impurities to the outside world.

I myself do a lot of juice cleansing. I try to do one hundred days per year. In fact, as I write this now, I am on my fiftieth consecutive day on nothing but juice and tea. I've done many fasts and feasts in my time, but this one is different because of experience. My mind is at a different level of training now, as the food addictions have melted away.

I feel great. I'm running five miles at a time, lifting weights, and doing yoga with no problems. *NOTE: I do not recommend anyone does this type of exercising while fasting unless they have experience. Yoga, walking, and swimming however, are exercises one should do when cleansing.*

This feast has been great research on not needing solid foods to thrive athletically. Most people are shocked when I tell them I haven't eaten in so long. They're like, "Oh my God, but you have so much energy!" Well, yeah, of course I do, because my body isn't doing much digesting and my cells are being fueled with tons of

SUNLIGHT. If one has an understanding of the human body, one will understand this level of health.

I'm starting a detox intensive soon with certain fruits and botanicals to clear my body. Coming off of this juice cleanse is going to give the body a huge head start and the fruits and botanicals are going to sweep and strengthen like never before. I'm expecting a few "healing crises" certainly.

I understand some view this as radical. Well, to me, eating movie theater popcorn or eating burgers and fries is radical. You see, even though I'm an expert on chronic illness and considered a "health guru" to many people, I myself have issues that need to be "fixed." This is my passion and my mission, because the more I work on me, the more I can help others.

I know because I do, while others think they know because they were told. You should be weary of who you listen to. Make sure they know because they do.

SOCIAL MEDIA ASSIGNMENT:

Post about your juice feast. How do you feel? How is your energy level? Are you noticing progress? Do you feel like you can climb mountains and run marathons? Are you having any detox symptoms? I want to know.

TAGS: #JuiceFeast #Detox #SunlightJuice #ThreeDLife #EatTheSunlight

---

BOTANICALS FORMULAS

Botany is the science of plants. Even long before humans started studying plants, we have been using them to heal. Many wild animals use them as well. There are herbs, roots, leaves, seeds, and more that come together to help us. With technological advancements in society, we can now create botanical formulas in the form of tinctures, capsules, or teas.

I think what herbalists do is amazing. They research what certain botanicals do, then they mix them together to create magic! Many refer to this method as "Chinese medicine."

Botanical formulas are a must for detox intensives. They clean, strengthen, and regenerate our tissues and cells. Each formula has a purpose. You can find formulas for kidneys, liver, lymph, brain, nervous system, and more. Again, find a specialist who can create an individualized protocol for you.

Here are some examples of botanicals used in formulas:

Licorice Root

Marshmallow Root

Burdock Root

Cat's Claw Bark

White Oak Bark

Milk Thistle

Fennel Seeds

Dandelion Greens

Chickweed Herb

Plantain Leaf

It's important to understand botanical formulas are not enough. You must be eating the proper diet. And of course, when detoxing, that diet is juicy fruit, fresh juices, or both.

DETOX INTENSIVE

A detox intensive consists of a high fruit or juice diet combined with an individualized protocol of botanical formulas for a longer period of time. A detox intensive is not short like a cleanse. It can be anywhere from three months to three years. It all depends on how much work you want to put in.

Through this ancient practice, we can revitalize the body as we purge out accumulated wastes, giving the tissue an opportunity to regenerate as the body reverses its malfunctions. This is the process used to help others achieve restoration from chronic illnesses, viruses, or cancers.

I'm sure a few of you reading this just jumped up and said, "Wow! I'm going to get rid of my illness by detoxing!" Hold on. While it is possible that you can do it on your own, I always recommend hiring a specialist to coach you through it. I tell clients all the time, "healing hurts." And it does (more on this later). It can get scary. This is why I started a division of chronic illness specialists on my website.

People may judge this method and ask, "When is enough?" or "Aren't you healthy already?" Well, think about how much damage we have done to ourselves from our food and beverage addictions. Now add in stress and genetics. My detox teacher, Robert Morse, ND, refers to your health choices as "hellville" and "wellville." You can either suffer in pain while living an artificial life, or you can put in the work and achieve vitality. Pick one.

When you go this deep on an intensive, it's important to make sure the second "D" is good too. You want to have a sound, stress-free mind when putting in this much work. This is another example of why the #ThreeDLife is so crucial for vitality.

HEALING HURTS

One of the phrases I use with clients is "healing hurts." You see, it's a given that when you are cleaning acids and waste, they're going to sting on the way out. When they're loosened from the tissue, they go back into circulation before being removed to the outside world. For example, if one did a significant amount of drugs (legal or illegal) in their life, these leftover toxins will create a pretty intense detox. Someone may even get high again as they're going through the process.

Detox symptoms come in the form of headaches, rashes, vivid dreams, a sore throat, and more. We must put in perspective that our whole lives we have consumed prescriptions drugs, additives, chemicals, hormones, and preservatives. It's important to keep track of these detox symptoms, because it exposes our weaknesses. Example: If you get a rash on your left leg consistently, that means you have a problem in that area.

When you're going hard and doing a detox intensive, you may have what we call a "healing event" or "healing crisis." I've seen people break out in a full body rash. I've seen people stuck on the couch with flu-like symptoms, and certainly many times, folks may have to go to the ER. For instance, if you had bronchitis on and off your whole life, it may happen again on a detox intensive. It could even evolve into pneumonia. If that were to happen, it just means you're healing. But when this happens, sometimes chronic becomes acute. When it becomes acute, you may need emergency care to help you through it.

The ER can be your friend in a detox intensive. Again, this is why you want to hire a specialist. That specialist will "walk the line" with you so you don't have to go to the ER. They can pull back on certain botanical formulas, take you off, or put you on certain foods. There is an art to a detox protocol.

There is no way around it: If you want to heal, you're going to have to go through the pain to restore the human body. It's just part of the deal. I think my clients want to punch me sometimes, because they will contact me and tell me about their toenail falling off, or coughing up blood, or having flu-like symptoms, and I will say, "congrats!"

The problem is, when someone with no experience is detoxing, they will get scared from the symptoms, and then they go back to their food of choice, which will suppress the symptoms. And by suppressing the symptoms now, they will see chronic or cancerous issues later. This is similar to detoxing folks with drug addictions. After a while, some drug addicts take the drug solely to stay "normal" because they're scared of the detox symptoms. If you take an alcoholic or drug addict off their attachment of choice, their withdrawal symptoms will be intense. That's why they have treatment centers for these things. Do you remember the scene in the movie *Ray* when Ray Charles (played by Jamie Foxx) was detoxing off of heroin?

If you're doing a detox intensive and have healing events, don't expect others to understand. They will call you nuts, and some will urge you to stop what you're doing. Your MD will too. He would rather give you meds so he can get a cut. This is what happened to a younger Steve Jobs when he went to the hospital from doing an all fruit diet. He was simply detoxing! He was healing himself. But because it made headlines, it gave fruit a bad name.

Sometimes a detox intensive could take away from your daily life. This should NOT discourage you from doing a detox intensive, for you can still make it work.

Just use your vacation and sick days at your job as needed. Again, if you have a specialist coaching you, that specialist can help you "walk the line" so you can still partake in your daily life. I do not recommend doing a detox intensive on your own.

TONGUE

When you're detoxing, especially juice feasting, pay attention to the color of your tongue. Pink is its natural color, but while you are in the process, it becomes greenish, brownish, or whitish. What's going on with the tongue gives you a pretty good idea of what is going on in the gut.

The coating will be thick and dark if you are very toxic. And of course, the thinner and lighter the coat, the cleaner you are. When you tongue returns to its natural pink color, it's an indication that you have done a great job of cleaning and you can stop. But you don't have to. You can keep going if you want to cleanse deeper.

#ThreeDLife
Success Stories

The #ThreeDLife allowed me to gradually make serious changes to important areas affecting my health: my diet, my stress management, and detoxification. I first tried the program after having surgery for endometriosis, and I was determined to never have surgery again. The program has changed my life, and I will never look at food, stress, and detox the same again. The program also helped me to realize areas of strength and weakness both mentally and physically and to understand myself in a completely different way. Everything I learned in the program was invaluable, and I am so glad that I took this important step to ensure my health and wellness. Coach Reese is extremely supportive, knowledgeable, and a great motivator. If you want to change your life for the better, try the #ThreeDlife.
-Nakia Hamlett

COLONICS & ENEMAS

A colonic is an alternative therapy that removes waste products from the colon by purging with purified water. This process doesn't get deep into the tissues, but certainly clears your pipes of anything that is loose. While many people (especially in the medical field) don't advocate colonics, I think they can be very useful. I believe that the key to get an effective colonic is all about when you get it done. I think there are three circumstances to get one:

1. When you're cleansing (fruit feast or juice feast)

2. If you're obese and making a diet change

3. If you're suffering from chronic constipation

I only get a colonic done when I'm cleansing. It makes sense because the fruit or juice feast has loosened up the toxins from the tissues, and then the purified water washes them away like a river. If you get a colonic while you're still consuming a poor diet, it serves not much of a point, as you will only be washing away a few days of food. I've gotten colonics done twenty days into a juice feast, and a lot came out. If I didn't eat solid food in twenty days, how could that much be removed? That is a deep and effective colonic!

If someone is obese, then I recommend finding a good colonic center and getting their largest package. This will help the obese person remove wastes and get a jump-start on losing weight.

However, I only recommend this if this person is in the process of changing their diet for the better. Otherwise, it makes no sense.

If you're constipated, then you need a colonic or enema immediately. You do not let wastes just hang out inside you for long periods of time. Not only is this horrible for your gut and colon, but it can cause chest pains and even heart attacks. Our bodies are not meant to operate with blockages.

As far as enemas go, they are smaller versions of a colonic, which can be done at home. They are very useful, and you should always have colonic bags on hand just in case. They are great for when you're juice feasting, so you can cleanse your colon every few days.

If you want to see an example of a colonic, I documented one of mine! It's on my YouTube channel. Enjoy! (This is a great part of the book where I break out some social media language.) LOL...SMH

SAUNAS & STEAM ROOMS

These are great tools that we can use to help remove some extra toxins. But make no mistake about it; they are far from the end all be all.

I spend a good amount of time in the sauna at my gym, and I hear guys all the time talk about removing their toxins. Especially on a Monday when they swear they are detoxing the food and alcohol they had over the weekend. While they technically aren't lying because they're detoxing by definition, it's far from the healing process that I'm talking about in this book.

Repeated use of a hot room slowly restores skin elimination, and toxic chemicals and metals can be removed fast. In fact, you may notice that you have red blotches on your skin when you get out of the sauna or steam room. Those are acids coming out, and guess what? They're not blue!

Raising the body temperature causes infections to heal more quickly and can help combat infections. This is why our bodies develop fevers when we're ill to enhance metabolism and help kill germs. It is also why we should not take anything for a fever unless your temperature hits one hundred four degrees. You want to sweat it out when you're sick. Again, your body is a living organism that knows what it's doing.

I recommend saunas and steam rooms, but make sure you hydrate before going in and especially when coming out. And please remember, it's just part of a cleansing; it doesn't replace fruit feasting, juice feasting, or an intensive protocol.

WHAT NOW?

I recommend cleansing around sixty days per year, and if you can, add in the sauna or steam room a few times a week.

Here are some cleansing options:

1. Perform a juice or fruit feast once per week (That's fifty-two days right there!)

2. Perform a month juice feast twice a year (i.e., January and July)

3. Perform a month fruit feast twice a year (i.e., March and September)

4. Perform six separate ten-day juice or fruit feasts throughout the year

While the detox intensive might not be something you feel you're ready for, you must still cleanse when living the #ThreeDLife! Clean your house and strengthen its foundation. Add your detox practice into your yearly routines. Think of it as a holiday! Detox takes patience and practice. It will not happen overnight; you have to keep at it year in and year out. Experience will prove valuable in years to come. Again, it's a process.

INTERVIEW WITH A HEALER

When I decided I wanted to become a health professional, I knew I wanted to study under Robert Morse. I remember saving up my money to go to his school and being so excited when I was able to take that trip to Florida.

Morse isn't just a naturopathic doctor; he is also a biochemist, an herbalist, an iridologist, and spent time working in the emergency room. His knowledge and skills are as well-rounded as I've ever seen in the realm of health and healing. His clinic is responsible for helping thousands of people reverse their suffering while the allopathic establishment treats symptoms with medicine and many times just make it worse. Morse is considered by many to be the greatest healer today, and it was an honor to learn under him.

During his class back in 2012, I was fortunate enough to interview Morse on camera. Because he is and was a big part of my transformational journey, education, and growth, I decided to transcribe part of that interview and share it with you. I hope you get out of it what I have.

KWR: In your forty plus years, how many times have you seen somebody come to you with horrible symptoms and they reversed those symptoms?

Morse: Can I say everyday? I'll tell you, we only lose a few, and those are most involved where they've had the chemo and radiation, and they let years of that damage pile up on them. Most of those we can save, but there are always a few people once in a while who are just too far involved. But I've never seen anything where you couldn't rebuild the tissue. It's a lot of work for some people; it really is. But we've demonstrated this for years. The total regeneration of the human body, from bringing quads out of chairs, to seeing MS people walking again...You've seen all that, and that's what we do. We go in and rebuild the human body. It's simple, everyone can learn it, and it's not as difficult as you think.

KWR: And the lymphatic system plays a huge role. Why does the mainstream not know about the lymphatic system, and why is everyone not trained in it?

Morse: That's a question I've looked at for a lot of years, because allopathically, you would assume that this is the one system they would know. And if you look at interstitial fluid, that's the fluid that flows around your cells, it's 25 percent blood; the rest of it is that interstitial lymphatic fluid and that deals with the corrosive side of chemistry. And it's the corrosive side of chemistry that breaks us down. It's the same chemistry that breaks down car paint, statues...the same kind of chemistry that LA deals with causing lung cancer. It's all the acidic side of chemistry. When it's inside, it causes inflammation or acidosis, and then the breakdown of the cell eventually. And you have to remove that to get well.

KWR: Can you explain to my readers how important fruit is? Because we're conditioned to think fruits and veggies. How important is fruit versus veggies?

Morse: I think fruit should be about 75 percent of your diet, and vegetables 25 percent. If you have serious tumors, cancers, or painful arthritis, you name it, you need to ingest about 100 percent fruits, berries, and melons for a few months, maybe up to six months to get this out of you. And the reason is, fruits have the highest energetic principles and the highest astringents. So, they not only turn on your electrical system, which helps everything move better, but they help clean the kidneys and move that lymph astringently. And being high base chemistry, it helps bring a balance to the acid side of chemistry, creating hydration.

KWR: And they taste great! What about the theory that we human beings are frugivores?

Morse: Yes! I believe that! I've spent a few years as you know analyzing the anatomy and physiology of all the vertebrates. And what species do we look the closest to? Primates! There is no question. And that's on the outside and especially the inside. We are frugivores, and when we eat like them, we think better, we feel better, we clean better, everything is better. We just don't eat enough fruit because we're out of the tropical zone.

KWR: So should we be living in Costa Rica and Florida?

Morse: Basically. Living in a high alkaline environment pushes your diet toward the acid side of the food chain. And that's the protein side. Protein destroys kidney tissue, gut tissue, creates high acidosis, and now we start having our problems. As you know, the kidneys control your gigantic sewer system, and people have to understand your lymph system is the body's sewer system.

KWR: So what about these guys that go to the gym and they are real diesel...I mean they're in shape, they can run, they can jump, they can lift...

Morse: For a while, and then they come in to me and they're heading toward dialysis because of that high protein intake. Some lose their kidneys. I see it in pro athletes; they come to me all the time. Full of rheumatoid arthritis and full of inflammation. You can get stronger on the fruits. After they start cleaning out, then they start building. But it's strength, like a monkey. We were talking about how a little monkey can rip a human apart. But we don't eat raw foods; we don't eat our foods as nature gives them to us. We say, thank you God for making us this nice apple, but I like apple pie better. No, no, no. We've got to start eating food as nature gives it to us. We don't have to cook it—it's already been prepared.

KWR: The fire of death. *The Essene Gospel of Peace*.

Morse: That's right. I love *The Essene Gospel of Peace*.

KWR: You can take a picture of somebody's eyes and see so much. Please explain to my viewers.

Morse: Well, there was a surgeon back in 1853 who discovered that through the fibers in the iris, you can tell the strength or weaknesses of the cells in your body, what tissues were involved (liver, pancreas, bowel, etc.), you can see the lymphatic system, the nervous system; you can see almost the whole body from the eyes. And it works all through the nervous system, which is the communication network to the brain. So when you have a problem in your body, that problem is translated through the nervous system in full living color. And your eyes will change to adapt, and we learned how to read the eyes. This is the best thing an allopath has ever done was discover iridology, because now we can see where you have that pain. We can see where you're suffering, and we see why you're suffering. And no CAT scan or MRI can do that in most cases. You have to have a tumor before you can really see something.

KWR: How much longer do you see yourself practicing, because forty plus years is a long time?

Morse: Well, Jenson had seventy-five years in the field. Most of us healers will always be there, at one level or another. But I would like to retire myself. That's why I'm training all of you guys!

KWR: This seems to be like your mortal mission. You're spawning off other practitioners—it's like a ripple effect.

Morse: Well, we have to change the consciousness on the planet. The allopaths are out of control; they're hurting way too many people, and all these babies are dying. There is no remedy for treatment-based thinkers. We have to move from treatment-based thinking to causative thinking. What's causing your tumors? What's causing your pain? And then address that!

Full Interview Can Be Seen on YouTube:

www.YouTube.com/KevinWReese

CHAPTER 6

IF YOU'RE READY...SAY I'M READY

BE THE EXAMPLE

Diet, De-Stress, Detox is the formula to reclaim your life. When you #EatTheSunlight on a regular basis, you create less waste and more flow of energy within. But diet is never just enough; you must effectively handle stress as it comes, and also let go of the emotional pain of the past. And lastly, it's essential to remove wastes from your body and effectively clean out stored toxins from your tissues. When you live the #ThreeDLife, you start unclogging the physical and emotional obstructions that have held us back from true health, happiness, and vitality.

It's time for you to begin that #ThreeDLife. With the world—especially America—getting sicker every day, it's someone like you who will change it. And you don't change it by standing on the top of the mountain and preaching the #ThreeDLife or #EatTheSunlight. No. You change the world by changing yourself!

When you change yourself, you become a role model. And in doing so, others around you will eventually be inspired to change themselves. I tell clients all the time, "Act like you want it." That basically means…don't talk it, walk it.

Let me be an example. I was nearly two-hundred fifty pounds, back and forth to the MD. I had insomnia, I was a workaholic, and my ego controlled my emotions. I was addicted to marijuana, cigarettes, and worst of all, food! Chronic issues were developing, and a few trips to the ER and eventually finding myself on heart monitors left me feeling defeated. Looking up at the mountain and seeing how far I had to climb was overwhelming. I, just like you, would start to second-guess myself, psyche myself out, and let my mind (driver) take over. But a fighter fights, and mountains are meant to be climbed! With the attitude of wanting to thrive and not survive, I set out on a j   to chase healthy and vitality. And while I was doing it, people paid attention to me, and my example spread awareness and gave hope to others. In turn, many improved their lives by watching me improve mine, and some of them even became my very first clients.

I want you to understand that living the #ThreeDLife will make you different than others around you. We are programmed to act, eat, and believe a certain way and YOU WILL stand out. In the first few months, you may want to stay away from restaurants and family cookouts, so you can avoid the pressure while you are trying to overcome your addictions. But don't go overboard and become a recluse. You need to live a "normal" life in an "abnormal" way. So get back out there to the restaurants and cookouts as soon as you know you are ready to be a leader. If you decide to do the #ThreeDLife *12-Week Jump-Start Program*, we will teach you how to navigate at restaurants and cookouts so you can still mingle with friends and family.

Of course your coworkers and loved ones will ask questions. Of course they will criticize you because they think you're eating too much fruit. Of course they will think you're crazy because you're doing some cleansing. Of course you will be considered weird because you don't go to the bar. Of course there will be the doubters who will say things like, "We've eaten meat since cavemen times" or "you need protein." Of course you will have others who don't care, who will say things like, "I'm going to die anyway, I want to live life to the fullest." And of course, your ego is going to want to fight back from all these questions and comments.

Don't do it! In fact, you can blame it on me if you want. Let me be the "crazy" one. Tell them you read my book, and you're trying it out. Or drop a gem about primates never having blood sugar problems. But don't get into a big debate: Just show and prove. Everything is for everyone every time. But it won't be long before you're getting compliments on your weight, your skin, and your eyes for shining. And when the compliments start coming in and they ask what you're doing differently, say, "I #EatTheSunlight and live the #ThreeDLife."

Accept that taking on the #ThreeDLife is going to make you a unicorn among horses. Be proud of your choices! Answer the questions with a smile. Bring a watermelon to the cookout and eat the whole thing! Even bring a sunlight dish for others to try. And under no circumstances, criticize or frown upon what others are eating. Let them walk their path. You're creating a better and more natural way of life for you and your family. I want you to spread awareness by being the example. By being a leader.

SOCIAL MEDIA ASSIGNMENT:

Post about how you're standing out, so me and the other people on the #ThreeDLife can support you. Are others asking you questions? Are others criticizing you? Did you get hit with the "too much sugar" comment yet? Is anyone praising you? Are you getting compliments? How are you dealing with being a unicorn among horses?

TAGS: #UnicornAmongHorses #ThreeDLife #EatTheSunlight

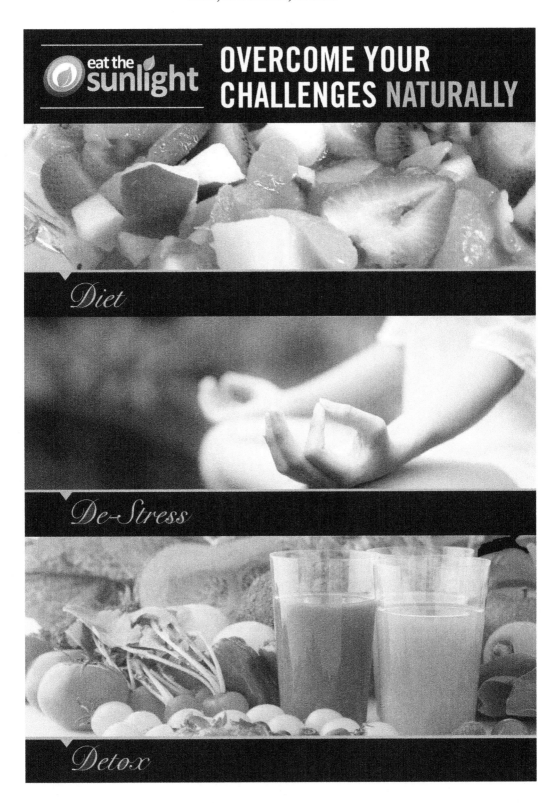

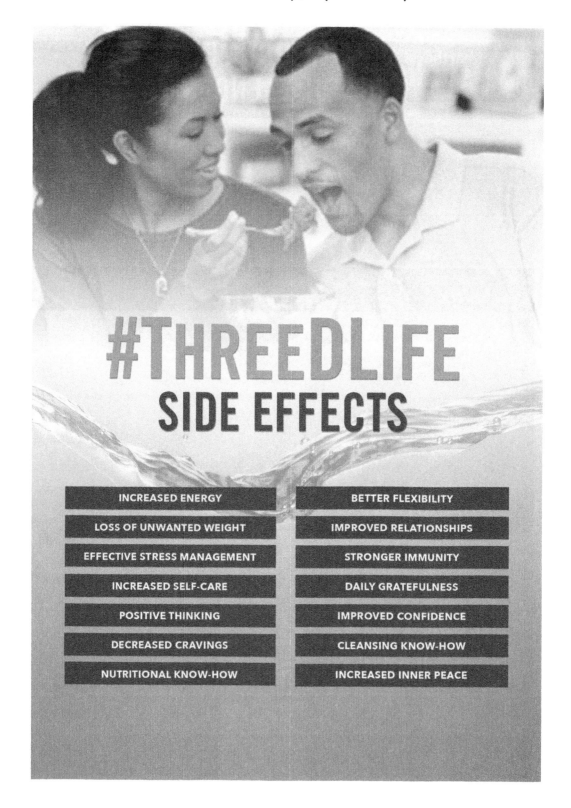

STEP UP TIME

And with all that said, I challenge you to step up! Try the #ThreeDLife for a few months and start fighting your programmed addictions. Eat the diet, practice the de-stressing, and cleanse your insides. Create balance inside yourself. Remember, It's not supposed to be easy. You will be a work in progress, just as I am.

SOCIAL MEDIA ASSIGNMENT:

Whether you have a chronic illness, you're obese, or you just know changing is the right thing to do, keep track of what happens over time! I want to see your results! Tell me! Show me! Even take a picture holding up the book!

TAGS: #KevinWReese #ThreeDLife #EatTheSunlight

We have plenty of recipes, videos, and blog posts on the website. Plus our weekly newsletter, which is sent directly from me. Plug in and let us motivate you! Once you feel confident in this new lifestyle, start taking your vitality test once per year and watch how each trip around the sun brings you closer to vitality!

If this book resonated with you, pass it to a loved one and be the example. You're a role model now. And believe me, as the world continues to get sicker…earthlings will need more people like you to inspire them. Congratulations, you just acquired a new purpose.

Now, if you're ready…say, "I'm ready!"

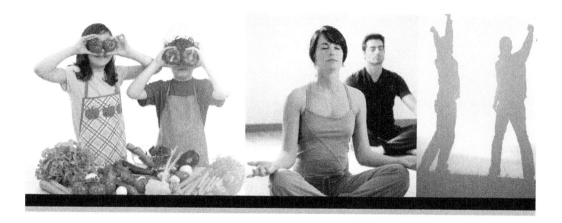

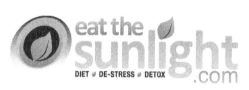

ABOUT THE AUTHOR

Kevin W. Reese is an author, motivational speaker, and health coach with an expertise in chronic illness. He's known for delivering a unique and powerful message by authentically blending education with entertainment.

As a sought-after public speaker, he's been invited to universities, high schools, festivals, children's events, and correctional institutions. A recording of his critically acclaimed seminar, *Root Cause: The Liberating Truth Behind Chronic Illness* was released as a fourteen-track album and his self-help book, *Diet, De-Stress, Detox: The Formula to Reclaiming Your Health & Vitality* has created a new trend in wellness.

Reese is a graduate of Eastern CT State University, the International School of Detoxification, the Institute for Integrative Nutrition, and is currently enrolled at the University of Natural Health working toward his Ph.D.

Before becoming a health professional, Reese was an unhealthy on-air personality at CBS Radio where he interviewed celebrities, hosted concerts, and was known as a "shock jock." A cigarette smoker with a severe food addiction, he eventually found himself on heart monitors at twenty-eight. Tired and fed up, he took control back by transforming his life with a holistic formula he created called the "Three D Life" (Diet, De-Stress, Detox). This resulted in losing nearly eighty pounds, quitting smoking, and reversing chronic issues. Through his shift, Kevin became passionate about natural health and followed his calling. Eventually, after a remarkable twelve years on the radio, he shocked his listeners by retiring from the airwaves to start his full-time health practice in 2012. Since then, he's helped others with arthritis, anemia, fibroids, diabetes, quitting smoking, and more.

MORE

TESTIMONIALS

"I've seen many speakers at expos and conferences regarding health, but Kevin is the only one I've seen that can touch the younger generation. It's a combination of his age, humor, and analogies. He can break barriers. His message is important."

- Nadia Smith

"I've traveled the world DJing, been on the road with Jadakiss, Mobb Deep, and recently, French Montana. I've always worked hard. I'm a workaholic, but I never put my health in order. A lot of my DJ buddies were going out and getting the surgery. I didn't have health insurance and didn't have the money for it. I was three-hundred and ten pounds, and now I weigh two-hundred thirty. Kevin stayed on me even when I didn't want to hear it. It just finally kicked in, and here I am eighty pounds later. I want to wholeheartedly thank Kevin for helping me change my life. The Sunlight works!"

- Mike "DJ Big Mike" Wilcox

"The Eat the Sunlight seminar was incredible. I've been vegan for thirteen years, and now it's so much clearer scientifically to me. All illness is caused by what you put in your body. It's a reality you either accept with hope, or deny for quick fixes to preventable problems that will never go away until changes are made."

- Joseph Cole

"Our cars come with an instruction manual; appliances come with instructions. Electronics and cameras come with instructional DVDs. EVERYTHING has a DVD, an insert, a pamphlet, instructions, diagrams, SOMETHING. I have put together shelving units, a swiveling TV stand, and even changed oil in a lawn mower. I just follow the instructions. Our bodies do not come with "how to" instructions, so we go through life blindly abusing our life force, our temple. For years, I have been starving my body, overeating at other times, and throwing all kinds of junk into it. Then I had a health scare. That was an eye opener, as it scared the crap out of me. We take for granted that our hearts will beat, that we don't have to think about taking breaths, and our blood will flow freely through our veins. We assume that's how everything in our body works until something fails,

then we are forced into preventative mode. Kevin W. Reese gave me the instruction manual for my body at a Sunlight Seminar. The good thing is that I can reverse conditions and heal myself. I just needed the directions. Now I feel enlightened. I understand how truly amazing my body really is. Thanks to Kevin, I know what I need to do to keep it functioning properly at its peak."

- Linda Reynolds

"I had such a great time at Kevin's Eat the Sunlight Seminar. I laughed until I cried. The examples that he used to break down what is happening in your body when you put bad things in it was educational. It was simple enough for everyone to grasp. I could definitely relate to a lot of things that he was saying, such as feeling like an outcast because of what you eat. It was nice to be around like-minded people and to listen to someone speaking with common sense and who had so much compassion for people's health."

- Shelby Ricks

"Amazing seminar with Kevin Reese. He has changed my view on food!"

- Janay Saxon

"Very educational, enlightening, entertaining, motivating, and inspiring seminar today! Thank you, Kevin W. Reese! Excited to start Eating more Sunlight!"

- Darla Blair

"Time to start eating more 'sunlight.' Thanks to Kevin Reese for the info at the seminar. I'm excited now about sunlight. Now I really know how great it is for me and my daughter. And I will increase our sunlight and hopefully my husband will follow along."

- Jeanette Vega

"If you are in the Southern New England area and can make it out here, I would strongly recommend it. Kevin is not only an inspiration to me as an entrepreneur, but as a human being, and his #EatTheSunlight movement is going to change healthcare as we know it! Anyone struggling with chronic illness (diabetes, lupus, cancer, etc.), at least check out his website if you can't make it! He has done a three-hundred sixty degree change in his own life, health wise, and is helping so many more! Check him out!!!"

- Lindsay Gilbert

"So just wanted to let you know your seminar/program has really inspired me. I've been trying to change my diet over the past week or so, and I really do like it. At least 85 percent of my diet has been fruits and vegetables since your seminar."

- Danielle Colon

"The East Coast's foremost authority on true detoxification and cellular regeneration, Kevin W. Reese is one of my favorite social media personalities. As someone who was left no other choice but to look outside of the allopathic (medical) community for solutions to autoimmune disease, I admire Kevin's creativity and dedication in helping those with chronic illness reduce suffering. His work has allowed me to reach new heights in my personal journey of fasting for health. A fantastic source of inspiration for those looking to realistically improve their dietary practice and overall lifestyle. Thanks for all you do!"

- Andrew Swalko

"I truly thank Kevin for providing me with knowledge at the Sunlight Seminar. It was amazing and easy to understand in every aspect. From learning the SUNLIGHT CODE to the writing exercise we did, Kevin might be some type of genius. I believe EAT THE SUNLIGHT will go worldwide. I'm still amazed."

- Jimmy Brunette

"After seeing Kevin make his transformation I was inspired. We had a real deep conversation and that gave me the spark I needed to change my life!"

\- Jorge Carrasquillo

"A couple of years ago, I was probably in the lowest and darkest part of my life. I was in college, dealing with a lot of personal issues, and my health was declining. I was on high blood pressure medicine, but I felt it wasn't making me any better and I was becoming increasingly depressed. One night, I began to watch a video with a guy wearing an 'Eat The Sunlight' shirt (who I later discovered was a man named Kevin W. Reese) interviewing some guy named DJ Big Mike and talking about how he lost seventy pounds and completely changed his life. About a year after I had started getting into eating healthier, my health was getting better, but my future was still uncertain. One day, I logged onto EatTheSunlight.com and saw that they were looking for an intern. My eyes lit up, and I applied right away, never thinking I would get lucky enough to get the position. As if some miracle had happened, I had gotten the call back that they wanted me, and I was then speaking on the phone with Kevin W. Reese, not knowing that this guy would impact me in the way that he did. Kevin is the type of person, that

even from the first time you talk to him, he makes you feel like he's known you for a long time. It made me feel good, since at that time I was having a lot of confidence issues, so I was beyond thankful to hear that he wanted me to start working with him. Working hard, he would always be there just to listen about any concerns I had as we talked about anything from wrestling to adrenal glands and even Jay-Z. About a year after our initial contact, I have completely gotten off of high blood pressure meds, graduated from college, gotten a job, am in the best shape of my life, and have been able to impact my family and friends as well. I wanted to take the time to write this letter of gratitude from the bottom of my heart."

- Jimmy Pierce

DIET, DE-STRESS, DETOX
QUIZ

1. Apes and humans are _____
A. Carnivores
B. Herbivores
C. Omnivores
D. Frugivores

2. What happens when you mix juicy fruit with other foods?
A. Headaches
B. Fermentation
C. UT Infections
D. Putrefaction

3. What is the only kind of fruit you can mix with other foods?
A. Citrus
B. Melons
C. Dried
D. Seasonal

4. Why shouldn't you drink liquid with your meals?
A. It dilutes the digestive enzymes
B. Causes gas
C. Causes blockages
D. Kills taste buds

5. The second most important food for a human is…
A. Potatoes
B. Greens
C. Protein
D. Quinoa

6. What system is the key to living sick-free?
A. Brain and nervous system
B. Circulatory system
C. Lymphatic system
D. Beta system

7. Which of the following is on the acid side of chemistry?
A. Water
B. Kale
C. Carbs
D. Protein

8. Organic produce has a 4-digit PLU# on the sticker?
True or False

9. If you have a rash, it's an indication that...
A. You need to poop
B. Your kidneys are not filtering properly
C. It's allergy season
D. You need to throw-up

10. Which of the following are considered healthy fats?
A. Walnuts
B. Avocado
C. Hemp Seeds
D. All of the above

11. A consistent high-protein diet creates...
A. Hair growth
B. Orgasms
C. Mucus and acid
D. Strong bones

12. Mixing protein with starches causes...
A. Headaches
B. Putrefaction
C. Fermentation
D. Dislocated earlobes

13. Which of the following is usually over four ingredients on its label?
A. Jarred olives
B. Canned beans
C. Apples
D. Bread

14. Why are berries the best for smoothies?
A. They taste great, and taste is all that matters
B. They're very important, and most people don't eat them because of their size
C. They tend to excite you in the morning
D. All of the above

15. A fruit smoothie is best for breakfast because you're breaking fast with the best food and emulsifying it so your digestive system doesn't get shocked.
True or False

16. When you blend blueberries and bananas together, you're making juice.
True or False

17. The #EatTheSunlight Diet is...
A. Fruits, vegetables, nuts, seeds, fish, beef

B. Fruits, vegetables, soda, fish, beef, seeds
C. Fruits, potatoes, fish, corn, nuts, seeds
D. Fruits, vegetables, nuts, seeds, herbs, sprouts

18. If you don't eat your uncooked sunlight…you didn't earn your one cooked meal for the day?
True or False

19. According to KWR, the root cause to people getting chronic illness is…
A. Milk
B. Chemtrails
C. Programming
D. Water

20. Medics and nurses can't remedy chronic illnesses; they are trained to treat acute or immediate issues.
True or False

21. What situation creates a fight-or-flight stress on the body?
A. Financial issues
B. Your boss yelling at you
C. Being chased by a lion
D. Getting ready for a date

22. Can you hold stress in your hand?
Yes or No

23. What part of the body is directly linked to stress?
A. Adrenal glands
B. Pancreas
C. Teeth
D. Ovaries

24. Someone tells you that you look great today. What does your "horse and carriage" say?
A. Ego triggers joy, and joy triggers a great feeling on the body
B. Memory triggers anger, and anger triggers a great feeling on the body

25. You have anxiety over driving in a snowstorm that is coming tomorrow…What does your "horse and carriage" say?
A. Memory triggers fear, and fear triggers anxiety on the body
B. Ego triggers joy, and joy triggers anxiety on the body

26. Ecstasy is as damaging as anger because it causes strong cravings, which can manifest into addictions?
True or False

27. In the "Interview With a Mystic," Nashid describes meditation as...
A. A car
B. A mirror
C. A cell phone
D. A radio

28. Your mind can be classically conditioned, just like a dog can be trained?
True or False

29. Who can sabotage you from staying with your goals?
A. Your significant other
B. Your child
C. Yourself
D. All of the above

30. You are obsessed with owning your own business, which you believe can make you a millionaire. This is your _____?
A. Ego
B. Pituitary gland
C. Memory
D. Adrenal glands

31. If you allow it to, annoyance will eventually turn to _____ then _____?
A. Joy, anger
B. Grapes, jelly
C. Anger, rage
D. Apples, juice

32. If you do visualization exercises with your mind, and picture something you want or need on a consistent basis, you will be putting that intention out into the universe.
True or False

33. What part of the mind does a craving for pizza come from?
A. Ego
B. Pineal
C. Memory
D. Center

34. Overthinking of the past can cause depression, and overthinking of the future can cause anxiety. So that means you want to practice living in the basement...

True or False

35. Hobbies are important because they are…
A. A way to lose weight
B. A life break with a purpose
C. A way to get depressed
D. All of the above

36. One of the great ways to practice "self-care" and stay positive is to….
A. Recognize your daily simple pleasures
B. Recognize the people who piss you off
C. Recognize all your faults
D. Recognize the cops on the highway

37. Holding resentment toward someone can cause hypersensitivity to everything they do or say.
True or False

38. It's possible to have gratitude for someone that you resent.
True or False

39. Stress contributes to illness by promoting lymphatic stagnation.
True or False

40. When in need of solitude and rest, the best place to go is…
A. The post office
B. The library
C. The zoo
D. The restaurant

41. No matter how healthy you live or think you live, toxins will enter your body through your foods, drinks, hygiene products, and air?
True or False

42. The three pillars of detoxification are…
A. Fruit feasting, juice feasting, and handstands
B. Fruit feasting, juice feasting, and massages
C. Fruit feasting, juice feasting, and botanical protocols
D. Fruit feasting, juice feasting, and protein shakes

43. When detoxing, fruit is the gas, and greens are the breaks?
True or False

44. When juice feasting, any feelings of hunger completely disappear after twenty-seven days.
True or False

45. A detox intensive consists of a high fruit or juice diet combined with an individualized protocol of _____ for a period of time.
A. Colonics
B. Oil pulling
C. Burgers and fries
D. Botanical formulas

46. When performing a detox intensive, it is possible to experience a _____?
A. Rash
B. Headache
C. Sore throat
D. All of the above

47. If you take an alcoholic or drug addict off their attachment of choice, their withdrawal symptoms will be easy.
True or False

48. KWR recommends everyone cleanses at least _____ days per year.
A. 1 day
B. 100 days
C. 10 days
D. 60 days

49. Performing a mono fruit feast over the course of a day is also called a _____?
A. Columbus Day
B. Monkey day
C. Crazy day
D. Cleaning day

50. The two fruits strongest for moving lymph fluid are…
A. Apples and grapes
B. Grapes and melons
C. Oranges and mushrooms
D. Melons and kiwi

51. If you want to do a detox intensive, you should hire a specialist.
True or False

52. An advantage of juice feasting is that it puts your _____ on a vacation.

A. Digestive system
B. Lymphatic system
C. Brain and nervous system
D. Beta system

53. In the "Interview with a Healer," Dr. Morse says that the acids in our bodies are the same chemistry that breaks down car paint, statues, and the same kind of chemistry that LA deals with causing lung cancer.
True or False

54. Looking at pictures of the eyes and seeing the fibers that indicate strength or weaknesses of the cells in your body is called _____ ?
A. Weirdology
B. Eye scans
C. Iridology
D. Window of the soul

55. You can detox while eating protein.
True or False

**Answers to the quiz are at:
www.KEVINWREESE.COM/THREEDLLIFEQUIZ

EXTRAS

KEVIN'S SEVEN RULES TO LIVE BY

1. Be Kind: Treat others how you want to be treated.

2. Be Healthy: Treat your mind and body as your sacred home.

3. Be Smart: Know because you do, not because someone told you.

4. Be Authentic: What others think of you is none of your business.

5. Be Safe but Strong: Confrontation is only necessary when it's necessary.

6. Be Happy: If you work on your passions and you're broke, you're still rich.

7. Be Resilient: The mountain is supposed to be steep, but the view is supposed to be seen.

KEVIN'S SEVEN BOOKS TO OWN & READ

1. *The Essene Gospel of Peace* by Edmond Bordeaux Szekely

2. *The Spiritual Notebook* by Paul Twitchell

3. *My Experiments With Truth* by MK Gandhi

4. *Love, Medicine & Miracles* by Bernie S. Siegel, MD

5. *Mucusless Diet Healing System* by Professor Arnold Ehret

6. *The Detox Miracle Sourcebook* by Robert Morse, ND

7. *The Celestine Prophecy* by James Redfield

KEVIN'S SEVEN FOODS TO EAT

1. Melons

2. Berries (includes grapes)

3. Apples

4. Peppers

5. Celery

6. Kale

7. Seeds

KEVIN'S SEVEN QUOTES

1. "We spend the first half of our lives making ourselves sick, and the second half of our lives trying to make ourselves un-sick." – Kevin W. Reese

2. "Don't just dip your toes in the water, do a running cannonball! If you belly-flop, get out of the pool, let the sting fade, then do another running cannonball! It's okay to belly-flop, just stop staring at the water. " – Kevin W. Reese

3. "The human body is a tube and tank machine with an electrical system that is made up of trillions of cells and two fluids, which are designed to create and react to chemistry. While this machine can malfunction, malfunctions can be fixed." – Kevin W. Reese

4. "Please explain to your children that fruit-loops and candy don't have real fruit in them. Feed them real fruit to teach them the origins of where a scientist got the idea from." - Kevin W. Reese

5. "In business, It's easy to get caught up in your competitive nature and lose sight on the person you want to be. But I'm learning that it's okay to be Kobe in the fourth. I don't mind taking the game over, throwing some elbows, talking a little trash and taking the last shot! But when the game is over, win or lose, I'm right back underneath the Bodhi Tree working internally. I feel protected and grounded. I am protected and grounded. And because of that…I always win, even when I missed that last shot." – Kevin W. Reese

6. "Something abnormal can become normal to you. Then you realize abnormal isn't normal and you are introduced to normal which feels abnormal. Normally this would be okay until you realize it's not normal." – Kevin W. Reese

7. "The world as you know it is only known by what you know. So if you strive to know more, you can change the world as you know it." – Kevin W. Reese

INTERVIEW WITH LUPE FIASCO

In 2012, as I was finishing up my last year as a radio personality, I had the chance to sit down with one of my favorite people to interview, outspoken rap artist Lupe Fiasco. During the interview, I decided to bring up nutrition.

KWR: Since we last spoke, I ended up going to nutrition school and became a health coach. I wanted to ask you, what role do you think nutrition plays in society right now?

Lupe: You mean the fattest country in the world? With a food network? Do you know what would happen if you put the food network in say, Ethiopia? Do you know what would happen to you? We're the fattest country on earth.

KWR: Why?

Lupe: Because we live in a manufactured, processed, high-fructose corn syrup world. All around fat, all around starch, potatoes with everything type of place. No real observations put on the benefits of vegetables.

KWR: The government spends no money promoting vegetables.

Lupe: Right, but it's not their job to tell you how to eat.

KWR: But they do with milk and meat though…

Lupe: Yeah, but it's not their job, they're just advising. It's an advisory council. But there's an economic thing to it. Just like there is an economic thing to grow vegetables. What I'm saying overall is, it's your job to dictate what you eat and what you put in your body.

This full interview is available on my old YouTube channel. www.Youtube.com/RunnindisRadio

Apple Rap
By Kevin W. Reese

Apples are best in the fall
but eat 'em year round, cuz they lower bad cholesterol

Please leave the milk alone
Apples got flavonoids and boron, this strengthens bones

If your asthma needs some easin'
Studies show that apple juice daily helps the wheezing

Whether it's when pain swells
or decreasing Alzheimer's by protecting your brain cells

Now I'm not saying that apples are the answer
But they do lower colon, liver, and lung cancer

Knocking out multiple opponents
And even protecting older women from osteoporosis

I say eat five of them, be a big eater
And don't forget to spare one for your teacher

Wait! I have one more amazing apple fact
There's no actual apples in Apple Jacks

See this video and more on my YouTube Channel
www.YouTube.com/KevinWReese

Parsley Rap
by Kevin W. Reese

Parsley is an herb that will help you be well
It's full of vitamin A, C, K and B12

It has antioxidants that neutralize smoke
And if you break it down to oils, it helps hair growth

It's great for all kinds of ear infections
And it stimulates kidneys to help hypertension

Ladies, if you're always moody and in poor zones
Call on parsley, it balances hormones

It should be a dream to ya
It supports iron absorption, making it great for anemia

It's even used to help with deafness
You should add it to your salad when at it's freshest

It even helps break down protein and fat
That's why they serve it with steak, you ever think of that?

So whether you're spicing up foods or using it for health
Parsley is an herb that was put here to help

See this video and more on my YouTube Channel
www.YouTube.com/KevinWReese

Cucumber Rap
By Kevin W. Reese

Of course the cucumber, it's a mighty good choice
A source of silica, it helps with pain in your joints

It's not from a root, a relative of the melon
It's got seeds, it's actually a fruit

With your skin, they're automatic
Helps wrinkles, cuts, puffiness, and rashes

It's time for you to think
Full of B vitamins, so you don't need that energy drink

Diabetes is dangerous
But cuk juice produces insulin from pancreas

Got bad breath? Well I got a weapon
Put a slice in the roof of your mouth for thirty seconds

Is your hair going bare slow?
Well if you care, they stimulate hair growth

So brighten up your salads at night
Or just wash it off, and take a bite

See this video and more on my YouTube Channel
www.YouTube.com/KevinWReese

Chronic Realness
by Kevin W. Reese

They say I'm a little different, first impressions of a guy
With a chain wallet and a hat cocked to the side

I grew up on Wu-Tang, KRS & Biggie
I don't apologize for having hip-hop in me

Forget my fashion, I'm a natural health nerd
Focus on my words, my truth, and my passion

Cuz when I'm on the microphone
I Shift your mind and that's why, I bring light to the unknown

They're wondering if SUN is really?
A true healer, when he comes off so fun and silly

I've got a stout past, Reese, is an outcast
And I'll outlast, critiques, and down fads

I may not be your favorite cup of tea
But you'll always see authenticity

If you like me, tell a friend to get on it and feel this
Let 'em know, KWR suffers from chronic realness

See this video and more on my YouTube Channel
www.YouTube.com/KevinWReese

THANK YOU

Mom and Dad, Kevin Wright, Jessica Mays, Chris Cabott, Nashid Fareed-Ma'at, Joe Lachance, Taylor DeWitt, Milo Sheff, Linda Larensen, Sarah Hatcher, Mike Wilcox, June Archer, Mike Vezzola, Tia Ingram, Buck Collins, Victor Star, Allan Garland, Joan Dillon, Nancy Barrow, Linda Reynolds, Mary Jones, Chris Wright, John Sheatsley, Stacey Downing, Walter McEntire, Annette Belzowski, Sarah Basile, Jorge Carrasquillo, Tunde Junior, Matthew Frenis, Karl Koenig, Eric Hollis, Craig Moore, Chad Bromley, Chris Fury, Ron Stewart, Felipe Rei, Eva Marie, Jimmy Pierce, Philip McCluskey, Glen Colello, Sarah Bamford, Marc and the whole Meli-Melo Café in Greenwich, Curt Griffing, Ami Beach, Anthony Canelo, The Robinson Family, Robert Morse, Dan McDonald, Kris Parker, Germaine Williams, and all my clients.

You have all helped me on my journey in some form or way.

Thank you!

PUBLISHED WORKS
By Kevin W. Reese

Diet, De-Stress, Detox:

The Formula For Reclaiming Your Health & Vitality

Root Cause:

The Liberating Truth Behind Chronic Illness

#Protein Kills:

Seven Reasons Why a High-Protein Diet Can Be Deadly

Available On

Amazon.com

KevinWReese.com

INDEX

dairy, 50, 83, 84, 110

denatured, 50, 53, 57, 60, 61, 69, 74, 92, 105, 118, 123

depression, 23, 147, 162, 268

DE-STRESS, 2, 127, 220

DETOX, 2, 19, 27, 28, 29, 30, 95, 117, 159, 168, 213, 215, 216, 217, 218, 220, 226, 227, 229, 230, 231, 232, 238, 263, 270, 271

detox intensive, 216, 229, 231, 232

DIET, 2, 219

digestion, 16, 29, 136

drama, 17, 134, 137, 139, 140, 141, 147, 175, 182, 205

edema, 22, 42

ego, 143, 146, 147, 267, 268

enzymes, 19, 69, 76, 93, 95, 100, 102, 105, 125, 222, 224, 264

fermentation, 93, 94, 264, 265

fibromyalgia, 5, 14, 21, 42, 201

fish, 23, 73, 85, 86, 109, 266

fitness, 20, 23, 26, 23, 44, 74, 198, 199, 200, 202, 203

flesh, 17, 21, 18, 33, 35, 37, 39, 48, 49, 51, 63, 69, 85, 86, 93, 94, 95, 103, 104, 105, 107, 109, 110, 120, 121, 168, 181

frugivore, 49

fruit, 49, 50, 52, 56, 58, 63, 66, 216, 217, 218, 269

genetics, 9, 6, 8, 9, 10, 11, 12, 230

glands, 7, 20, 4, 35, 36, 37, 38, 57, 120, 125, 213, 267, 268

glycemic load, 58

GMO, 18, 74, 79, 80

gratitude, 188, 189, 190, 191

herbivore, 33

herbs, 38, 60, 78, 92, 95, 105, 107, 118, 124, 125, 227, 266

HIIT, 199, 200, 202, 203, 204

immune response, 21, 60, 71, 74, 92, 105

insomnia, 138, 201

juice, 66, 113, 216, 219

kidneys, 14, 15, 25, 27, 28, 32, 71, 72, 214, 227, 241, 242, 265, 279

NOTES

www.EATTHESUNLIGHT.com

www.KEVINWREESE.com

Write to KWR

PO Box 380261

East Hartford, CT 06138

Lightning Source UK Ltd.
Milton Keynes UK
UKOW05f2114020915

257981UK00005B/112/P